T0222225

Calm and Confident Under Stress

Gert Kaluza

Calm and Confident Under Stress

The Stress Competence Book: Recognize, Understand, Manage Stress

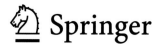 Springer

Gert Kaluza
GKM Institute for Health Psychology
Marburg, Germany

ISBN 978-3-662-64439-3   ISBN 978-3-662-64440-9   (eBook)
https://doi.org/10.1007/978-3-662-64440-9

This Springer imprint is published by the registered company Springer-Verlag GmbH, DE, part of
Springer Nature.
The registered company address is: Heidelberger Platz 3, 14197 Berlin, Germany

Preface

Dear Reader,

As the author of this book, I welcome you very warmly. I am pleased about your interest.

For more than 25 years now, I have been dealing with the topic of "stress and stress management" as a researcher and teacher as well as a trainer and coach. This book represents my attempt to summarize the knowledge and experience gained in an understandable language and practical for a wider audience. It tries to build a bridge between scientific-theoretical foundation on the one hand and practical application on the other. I hope that this balancing act between theory and practice has been successful.

Over the past three decades, interest in the topic of stress has steadily increased both among experts and the general public. The reasons for this are, on the one hand, serious changes in our living and working conditions, which lead to stress for more and more people. On the other hand, recent findings in neurobiological and health science research have deepened our understanding of stress and its significance for the health of the individual. Both developments will be discussed in this book.

My own continuing interest in the subject is based not only on its great significance for health, but also on the fact that in stress events, it can be seen particularly impressively how social conditions, individual experiences and behaviours, and biological processes are closely interconnected. In stress, we always react as a whole person with heart and muscles, with feelings and thoughts, and with typical actions. Stress requires a holistic approach from different perspectives. In this book, I would like to introduce you to such a comprehensive view of the stress phenomenon.

It is my conviction that understanding is a necessary prerequisite for effective action. In this respect, I have endeavoured in the first part of this book to present the social, psychological, and biological processes that determine the occurrence of stress in a comprehensive and at the same time comprehensible manner. The second part of the book then deals with possible courses of action for dealing with stress. It is not my intention to provide you with simple advice and patent remedies. Because these do not really exist. Instead, I would like to show you a wide variety of possible courses of action and encourage you to find your own individual way of dealing calmly and healthily with stress at work and in everyday life. I am deeply convinced that not only we are victims of stressful circumstances to which we are helplessly exposed, but also each individual has external and internal freedom, decision-making possibilities, and room for manoeuvre to take care of his or her own physical and mental well-being despite existing external stressors. It is my hope that such a conviction will grow in you as you read this book and that you will find the courage to recognize and use your freedom.

This is the 7th edition of the book. The 1st edition was published in 1991. After the text was completely revised and brought up to date for the previous 6th edition of this book, I have only made a few necessary error corrections in this 7th edition. This book is written first and foremost for all stress-ridden people: for people who already feel the first physical or mental signs of overload or incipient exhaustion, for people who suffer from illnesses in whose development or in whose course stress also plays a role, and of course especially for all those who do not want it to get that far in the first place and want to develop their stress competence. Furthermore, the book addresses people who are entrusted with personnel responsibility in their profession: managers in business and administration, specialists from human resources and personnel developers, trainers, and generally teachers and educational professionals. This book is also written for professionals in healthcare, rehabilitation, social work, and social pedagogy and for therapists and counsellors who deal with stressed patients and clients in their daily work.

I wish you an informative, stimulating, and hopefully motivating read. I look forward to your suggestions, constructive feedback, and experience reports. Write to me at info@gkm-institut.de.

I would like to thank the staff of Springer Verlag for their professional support of the book over many years, especially Monika Radecki, Sigrid Janke, and Barbara Buchter (editing).

Gert Kaluza
Marburg, Germany
September 2022

Contents

II   Coping with Stress

About the Author

Gert Kaluza

is a psychological psychotherapist and works as a trainer, coach, and author in the field of individual and workplace health promotion. After working at various universities for over 20 years, he founded his own further education and training institute in 2002 (▶ www.gkm-institut.de). He is married, father of three adult daughters, and grandfather of several grandchildren. He finds his own balance in running in the woods, on the golf course, and with the Tango Argentino.

GKM Institute for Health Psychology, Marburg, Germany

Recognizing and Understanding Stress

Contents

Stress: What Is It Actually? An Introduction

Contents

© Springer-Verlag GmbH Germany, part of Springer Nature 2022
G. Kaluza, *Calm and Confident Under Stress*, https://doi.org/10.1007/978-3-662-64440-9_1

1

Stress in science

Stress—hardly anyone knew this word 50 years ago. At most, a few material scientists used it to describe physical forces that act on solid bodies and deform them under certain circumstances. In the 1940s, the Austrian-Canadian physician and biochemist Hans Selye (1907–1982) introduced the concept of stress into medicine. He used it to refer in general terms to the effects of stress on living bodies. His research showed that a wide variety of physical and mental loads lead to characteristic physical and mental changes that, if prolonged, can pose a serious threat to health. Scientists from different disciplines such as biology and medicine, psychology, sociology, and occupational science have since intensively researched the development of stress and its consequences for physical and mental health.

Stress as a health risk factor

Today, there is no longer any doubt that stress is one of the most important health risk factors people face in modern Western societies. The issue is also receiving increased attention on the political stage. For example, the European Agency for Safety and Health at Work stated as early as 2000 that work-related stress is one of the greatest threats to the well-being of employees. Europe-wide surveys have shown that almost one in three workers is affected. Studies suggest that 50–60% of all lost working days are related to stress problems. Trade unions are calling for legislators to introduce "anti-stress legislation". Human resources managers in companies are increasingly confronted with the question of how they can maintain and promote the performance of employees in the long term in the face of an ageing workforce and increasing psychological pressure.

Stress in politics and society

So it is not surprising that the concept of stress has now found such a pervasive entry into everyday language as probably few terms from science. There is talk not only of stress at work but also of stress at school and even in kindergarten. There is performance stress, relationship stress, and even leisure stress, right up to stress in hospital, in traffic, and even on holiday. There is hardly an area of everyday life that is not associated with this term. Stress—it seems—rules our lives. "I'm stressed!" or "I'm under stress!" are frequently voiced and heard responses to the question of personal well-being. Stress is also increasingly used as an explanation for a wide variety of impairments to physical and mental well-being ("It's the stress"). And sometimes, the remark "I'm under stress!" is also used to excuse one's own misconduct to oneself and others and to avoid a critical discussion with oneself and others.

Stress in everyday life

Finally, it is not uncommon for an undertone of pride to be mixed into the complaint about too much stress. Here stress becomes a sign of the importance and significance of one's own person, a status symbol that promises recognition from others.

■ **But What Is Stress Anyway? What Triggers It and How Does It Manifest Itself?**

In this introductory chapter, I would like to begin by clarifying the understanding of stress that underlies today's modern science and that will also form the basis for our later considerations of starting points and strategies for stress management. I will outline a simple framework model that will help to distinguish essential aspects of the stress event and to identify possible starting points for stress management.

1.1 The Stresstrias

Herbert M., in his mid-40s, works as a senior engineer in a large construction company. He is married and has three school-age children. He has been under constant professional strain for 2 years now. Internal restructuring, the introduction of new computer-aided design processes and, last but not least, the success of his company on the market have led to an ever-increasing workload and increasingly demanding requirements. His colleagues regard him as ambitious and enthusiastic. His boss appreciates his sense of responsibility and his eagerness to work, and this recognition is enormously important to him. He does not really know when to call it a day and prefers to take care of everything himself before relying on others. For some time now, family worries have also been weighing him down. His father, who is in need of care and who also lives in the household, is becoming increasingly difficult, and his wife demands more support and accuses him of not caring enough for the family. Herbert M. increasingly feels that everything is getting on top of him. Although he works longer and longer hours in the evenings and also takes work into the weekends, he manages less and less. He has trouble concentrating. At night, his thoughts circle and he finds it difficult to sleep. During the day, fatigue, headaches, nervousness, and irritability are already the norm. Sometimes, he feels pains in his chest that frighten him.

An example

In every stressful event—as in Herbert M.'s example—three aspects can always be distinguished from one another. Before you continue reading, please take a moment to reflect on your own personal experience of stress (▶ Box 1.1).

How do I experience stress?

Box 1.1: Stimulating Self-reflection: Stress—What Is It Actually?

Please take a moment to reflect on your own personal experience of stress recently. The following three sentence starters should help you to organize your thoughts. Please complete

1

each of the three sentences as it corresponds to your personal stress experience.
- I get stressed when...
- When I'm stressed, then...
- I'm putting myself under stress by ...

Here are some common and typical expressions of other people:

I get stressed when...
- several things have to be done at the same time.
- different people want different things from me, and preferably at the same time.
- I get criticized.
- disruptions and interruptions throw off my schedule.
- my e-mail box is overflowing.
- the day begins with a rush in the morning.
- I can't resolve an argument with others.

When I'm stressed, then ...
- I get clammy hands, dry mouth, heart palpitations, a lump in my throat, stomach aches, and neck tension.
- I have trouble sleeping.
- I get all hectic and nervous inside.
- I have trouble concentrating and lose track of things.
- I fly off the handle and raise my voice.
- I smoke more than normal.

I'm putting myself under stress by ...
- I want to do everything 150%.
- I'm taking on too much.
- I make daily schedules that are impossible to manage at all.
- I always want to please everybody.
- I don't give myself a break.
- I care too much what other people think about me.
- I want to take care of everything myself.

Stress consists of three parts

Stressors

You will have noticed that the three sentence beginnings each highlight different aspects of the stress event. These are the three components of stress, which must always be distinguished when we talk about stress (◯ Fig. 1.1).

The first sentence beginning *"I get stressed when ..."* is aimed at the triggers of stress in the form of external stressful conditions and demands. We also call these **stressors**. In the case of Herbert M., these are above all the increased demands at work as well as his father's increasing need for care and the conflict with his wife that is developing over this.

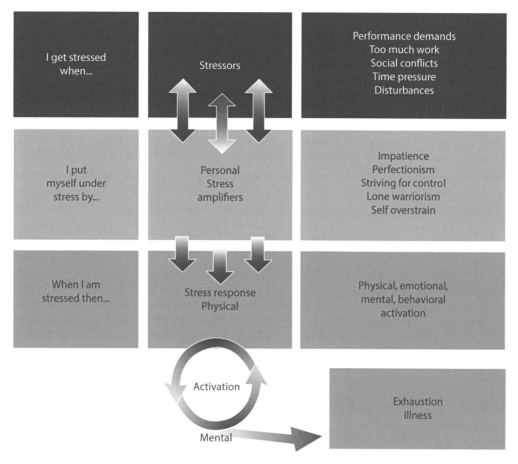

◘ Fig. 1.1 The three components of the stress event

The second sentence beginning *"When I am stressed, then ..."* is aimed at what happens in us and with us when we are confronted with stressors. We are therefore concerned here with the physical and psychological responses to stress. We refer to these accordingly as **stress reactions**. Herbert M. shows typical stress reactions such as increasing nervousness, irritability, and lack of concentration as well as headaches, sleep disorders, and heart complaints.

Finally, the third sentence, *"I put myself under stress by ..."*, addresses personal motives and inner attitudes with which we approach stressful situations and which are often decisive in determining whether stress reactions occur at all and how strongly they turn out in these situations. These personal motives and attitudes shape personal stress processing and, to a certain extent, represent the links between the external stressful situations (the stressors) and the stress reactions. We refer to them as **personal stress amplifiers**. Personal stress

Stress response

Personal attitudes as stress amplifiers

1

intensifiers that play a role in Herbert M.'s case are, above all, his strong need for recognition, especially at work, and his desire to do everything himself if possible. Other frequent personal stress intensifiers are perfectionist demands for performance and the desire to please everyone as much as possible.

Now let us take a closer look at these three aspects of stress.

1.2   Stressors: What Stresses Us Out

As already mentioned, we generally refer to stressors as all the conditions in our environment that trigger a stress reaction. These can be completely different situations such as a natural disaster, a car accident, a perceived unfair assessment by a superior, an overflowing e-mail inbox, a difficult customer meeting, a dispute in the neighbourhood, or a misplaced front door key.

Different types of stressors

Stressors can arise in the physical environment, for example, in the form of noise, intense heat or cold. Our own body can also become a source of stressors. Prime examples of this are pain, especially chronic pain conditions. Hunger and thirst, restricted movement, or itching can also trigger stress reactions. For many of us, mental stressors related to performance demands are at the forefront of the stress experience. Exams are just as much a part of this as constant time pressure, too many or too difficult tasks, or a high level of responsibility. In addition to performance stressors, social stressors, i.e. demands that arise in interpersonal contact, play a prominent role. Unresolved, smouldering conflicts with other people, competitive situations, but also isolation and especially experiences of separation and loss are examples of such interpersonal stressors.

Not every demand is a stressor

However, not every demand represents a stressor, that is not every demand automatically leads to physical and mental stress reactions. This is only the case with those demands where we are uncertain whether we will be able to cope with the demand. As long as we are certain that we can cope with a given challenge, we may have to make a great effort, but we will not experience stress.

This is particularly obvious and easy to understand in the example of an exam that we have to or want to take. This often becomes a stressful experience precisely because we are not sure whether we will be able to meet the requirements set. Without this subjective uncertainty about whether our own abilities will be sufficient, we are unlikely to experience stress in an examination situation, but may even regard it as a welcome opportunity to demonstrate our knowledge and skills.

Stress, therefore, always arises when there is a discrepancy between the demands and our coping skills. The experience of stress is all the more intense the higher the demands are assessed in relation to our own ability to cope. The decisive factor for a correct understanding of the stress experience is that it is based on the subjective assessment of the demands and one's own abilities and resources. It does not matter whether the situation in which we currently find ourselves is "objectively" seen or viewed from the outside as an excessive demand. The only decisive factor is that we experience and interpret this situation in this way. For the strength of our own stress experience, it ultimately does not matter whether our assessments correspond to reality or whether we overestimate the demands and underestimate our own abilities, for example, due to false expectations, too high demands on ourselves, or a lack of previous experiences of success.

The subjective assessment of requirements is decisive

The example of the exam also makes it clear that the more significant it is for us to successfully master the respective requirement, the more intense the stress experience. It makes a considerable difference to the degree of stress whether it is the all-important final exam or the monthly test for learning control. Significant means that successfully coping with it is important for us in terms of pursuing our own motives and goals. In the case of the exam, for example, it is about achieving educational and professional goals, but often also about maintaining and strengthening our own self-esteem or gaining emotional recognition from third parties. Stress arises when we see important goals and motives threatened. Here, too, it is ultimately not a question of the "objective" significance of the situation in question. The only thing that determines how intense stress is experienced is the importance we attach to the situation against the background of our own goals and motives and how threatening we subjectively assess a possible failure in this situation.

Stressors threaten personal goals and motives

Can you still remember your driving test? Did you also "sweat blood and water" back then? What is the source of the strong stress reactions that many young people experience in this situation? It is probably not so much the objective difficulty of the test requirement as the great subjective significance that obtaining a driving licence has for them. It is, in a sense, a symbol of entry into adulthood, promises new freedoms, and is of enormous importance to adolescent self-esteem. And how great would be the embarrassment in front of their peers, in front of their parents, and also in front of themselves if they were to stumble at this important developmental step!

Example "Driving test"

The example of the driving test points us to further characteristics of stressors that influence the strength of the stress

Transparency and control

1

reactions they trigger. As in the case of the driving test, it is in particular new, unfamiliar situations as well as situations that we ourselves cannot or can hardly influence or control, and situations that are poorly predictable or difficult to see through, that lead to stress reactions. Conversely, this also means that stress reactions can be reduced if, for example, there is a high level of transparency for employees at workplaces by means of clear specifications and information, and if employees are given their own opportunities for control and scope for action wherever possible.

Exams are only one example of stressors from the performance area. The explanations can easily be transferred to other performance-related and social demands, such as conducting a difficult customer meeting, preparing a project report, a balance sheet, or other work with a deadline, an unpleasant argument with a neighbour or the time-consuming care of a sick relative. Any of these demanding situations can trigger stress reactions, and they do so whenever we see personally significant goals and motives threatened and are uncertain whether our abilities will be sufficient to successfully cope with the demands at hand. In ▶ Chap. 3, we will look in more detail at the various forms of stressors in the world of work and in everyday life that are at the forefront of many people's experiences of stress today. At this point, we first note:

> **Conclusion**
> Stressors are demands whose successful management we assess as subjectively significant but uncertain.

1.3 Stress Response: Responses at All Levels

In stress the whole person reacts

The term stress reaction is used to describe all the processes that are set in motion on the part of the affected person in response to a stressor, that is everything that happens within us and to us when we are confronted with a stressor. Stress reactions show themselves in many ways on the physical level. They manifest themselves in observable behaviours by which outsiders can tell that someone is under stress, and they also affect the way we think and feel. We always react, so to speak, as a whole person with heart and muscles, with words and actions as well as with feelings and with thoughts to the confrontation with a stressor.

Stress mobilizes physical energy

On the **physical level**, stress leads to a multitude of changes that cause an overall physical activation and mobilization of energy. This can be felt, for example, in a faster heartbeat, increased muscle tension, or faster breathing. The physical stress reaction puts us in a state of readiness to act within a very short time. However, if this activation reaction is maintained over a longer period of time because stressors persist or recur, this gradually leads to states of exhaustion and to long-term negative consequences for health. What happens in detail and how the physical stress reaction can become a danger to health will be explained in detail in ▶ Chap. 2.

The second level of the stress response includes the so-called **overt behaviour**, what outsiders can observe. In other words, everything the person does or says in a stressful situation. Common stress behaviours include:

Typical behaviour under stress

- Hasty and impatient behaviour, for example, gulping down food quickly, cutting breaks short or skipping them altogether, speaking quickly and choppily, interrupting others;
- Narcotic behaviours, for example, smoking more and uncontrollably, eating or drinking alcohol or coffee, taking pain medications, sedatives, or stimulants;
- Uncoordinated work behaviour, for example, doing several things at once, "throwing oneself into work", lack of planning, overview and order, misplacing, losing or forgetting things;
- Motor restlessness, for example, drumming with fingers, scratching, nibbling at clothes, scuffing feet;
- Conflicting interactions with others, for example, aggressive, irritable behaviour towards family members, frequent disagreements over trivial matters, blaming others, rapid "going off the deep end".

The **cognitive-emotional level** of the stress reaction comprises the so-called hidden behaviour, inner psychological processes that are not directly visible to outsiders. In other words, all thoughts and feelings are triggered in the affected person in a stressful situation. Common cognitive-emotional stress reactions are, for example:

Typical feelings and thoughts under stress

- Feelings of inner turmoil, nervousness, and being rushed,
- Feelings and thoughts of discontent, anger, rage,
- Fear of failing, embarrassment, for example,
- Feelings and thoughts of helplessness,
- Self-blame and guilt,
- Circling, "brooding" thoughts,
- Emptiness in the head ("blackout"),
- Blocks to thinking, lack of concentration, "fluttering" thoughts,
- "Tunnel vision".

Often the physical, behavioural, emotional, and mental stress reactions build up on each other, so that the stress reactions

1

are reinforced or prolonged. A vicious circle can develop, for example, by uncontrolled acting out of the anger ("anger about the anger"), by fear of the physical stress symptoms ("fear of the fear") or struggling with the situation, one gets further and further into the stress-related excitement. However, it is also possible to have a beneficial mutual influence in the sense of dampening stress reactions. For example, we can reduce physical stress reactions through a relaxation exercise or through sport, and often cognitive and emotional calming can be initiated as a result. Just as, conversely, physical agitation can also be reduced, for example, through an emotionally relieving conversation.

We will deal in detail with the processes underlying physical stress reactions and their longer-term effects on health in ► Chap. 2. Let us note up to this point:

> **Conclusion**
> Stress reactions cause a general activation, which shows itself in characteristic changes of physical functions, of thoughts and feelings and in behaviour.

1.4 Personal Stress Amplifiers: Home-Made Stress

Stress is individual

Personal stress amplifiers in the form of individual motives, attitudes, and evaluations contribute to the fact that stress reactions are triggered or intensified. To a certain extent, they represent our "own share" in the stress event. Even everyday observation teaches us that different people respond to one and the same situation (e.g. an exam, an argument, a traffic jam, or a misplaced house key) with stress reactions of varying intensity. What drives one person up the wall, leaves another cold. Where one suffers from fear of failure, the other senses his chance. What one person feels particularly challenged by, another may withdraw from in resignation. Agreement on what is danger and what is not will only arise from person to person where there are extremely dangerous or even life-threatening circumstances. In the reality of everyday life, however, most assessments of how threatening a performance-related, interpersonal, or other everyday situation is vary widely from person to person. The reason for these differences is that the evaluation of a new situation depends on our respective personal previous experiences, which shape our expectations and fears, our motives and goals, our demands on ourselves, and on others.

A pronounced striving for profile, perfectionism, impatience, and especially the inability to accept one's own performance limits are widespread examples of such personal stress amplifiers. The idea of being indispensable oneself and a "lone wolf mentality" that does not allow one to accept support from others often add to the stress. In interpersonal situations, the desire to please everyone, an excessive striving for harmony, and a (too) strong dependence on the attention of others often contribute to the intense experience of stress. Sometimes stress is also used to avoid unpleasant mental realities that one does not want to admit. We put ourselves under pressure to avoid inner emptiness, depressive moods, feelings of meaninglessness, and loneliness. Stress thus becomes a means of escape from oneself.

Common personal stressors

These personal stress amplifiers form the individual background, which has grown in the course of our biography, against which we evaluate current demands in everyday life and work. They represent the glasses with which we go through our everyday life and with which we perceive and assess demands. Since these glasses are so much a fixed part of ourselves, it is often quite difficult to recognize and acknowledge their stress-increasing effect. Our own view of things appears to us as the only possible and correct one. What is needed here is the courage and the ability to distance ourselves from ourselves, so to speak, and to critically question ourselves.

Question personal stress amplifiers

Let us take some examples: If you are rushing through your everyday life under time pressure, do the causes really always and exclusively lie in the external deadlines set by others? Or do your personal impatience or the desire to do as much as possible at once also play a role? Would you get stressed after your superior has assigned you a new task, perhaps even saying that he needs a particularly capable employee for it? If so, are the causes of your stress solely due to the "objective" difficulty of the new task, or do the perfectionist demands you place on yourself and the unconditional desire not to disappoint your boss's expectations also play a role? Are you one of the increasing number of people who subject themselves to the dictates of the new communication media, who keep themselves available to others around the clock and who are thus unable to switch off properly in a state of permanent tension? Then ask yourself to what extent this constant accessibility actually corresponds to the requirements at work, for example, and to what extent your personal desire to be noticed and perceived as "important", or the desire to have everything under control yourself as much as possible, or the fear of missing out on something, also play a role.

It is often really not easy to tell the difference: Is *the stress coming from outside or am I putting myself under stress?* All too

Stress from outside or inside?

1

easily we are inclined to look for the causes of our stressful experience solely in external circumstances or in the behaviour of other people. In my seminars on stress management in the workplace, participants often report in detail about the increasing workload in companies, about poor organization or inadequate communication between superiors and employees. There is then a lot of complaining and accusation and also a feeling of helplessness and being at the mercy of others. Of course, these external stress factors play an important role in stress. However, the extent to which we are put under pressure by the above-mentioned workloads, the intensity of our physical stress response and our feelings of stress, in short, the extent to which we allow ourselves to be stressed, also depends to a large extent on how we relate to these stressors, how we assess them and our own possibilities for coping with them.

In ▶ Chap. 4 of this book, we will take a closer look at some of these personal stressors and their respective backgrounds. Let us note at this point:

> **Conclusion**
> Personal stress amplifiers are based on individual motives, attitudes, and evaluations that contribute significantly to triggering and/or amplifying stress reactions.

1.5 Stress Competence: From Victim to Actor

Acting instead of reacting

The basic understanding of stress on which I base this book assumes that every everyday stress event always involves an interplay of external stress factors on the one hand and internal personal stress intensifiers on the other. In order to get to the bottom of personal stress in everyday professional and private life, it is therefore crucial to clarify the relative importance of external stressors and internal stress intensifiers for the experience of stress in a specific situation (▶ Box 1.2). The question that needs to be asked and answered is: To what extent is the stress in this situation coming from outside and to what extent am I putting myself under stress? This seemingly simple question is a tough one. It requires courage and the willingness for critical self-reflection.

> **Box 1.2: Thinking Ahead: Getting to the Bottom of Stress**
> Please remember a typical stressful situation that you have experienced recently. Keep in mind as clearly as possible what happened and how you reacted to it. And then ask yourself:
> To what extent is the stress in this situation coming from outside and to what extent am I putting myself under stress?

Acknowledging the personal side of stressful events is often difficult for some people because they inwardly equate it with an admission of guilt, which then leads to feelings of incompetence and failure or even self-reproach. But this is a misunderstanding. It is not about personal guilt and individual failure. Rather, recognizing our "own share of stress" frees us from our experienced one-sided dependence on external circumstances. All too often we experience ourselves too one-sidedly as victims of the external stressors to which we find ourselves helplessly at the mercy. Instead of acting, we only react. The confrontation with our personal stress aggravating attitudes and behaviours opens our eyes to the free spaces, to decision-making possibilities and to the scope of action we have to take care of our own physical and mental well-being despite existing external stresses. With this book, I would like to give you suggestions and encourage you to recognize and use your freedom. Simple patent remedies and quick advice, however, do not really help here. Stress is a highly individual event, in terms of all three of its components: the stressors, the stress reactions, and the personal stress amplifiers. Accordingly, the approaches to stress management must be individual, related to the personal life and work situation and to the individual personality, in order to be successful in the long term. In the following chapters, I therefore first invite you to identify and understand your personal stressors, stress reactions, and stress amplifiers. In the second part of this book, I will then introduce you to the three pillars of personal stress competence and show you ways in which you can develop your own personal anti-stress strategy (◘ Fig. 1.2).

Patent remedies do not help

1

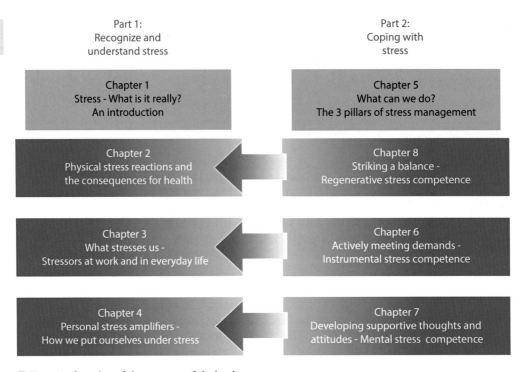

Fig. 1.2   Overview of the structure of the book

Physical Stress Reactions and the Consequences for Health

Contents

© Springer-Verlag GmbH Germany, part of Springer Nature 2022
G. Kaluza, *Calm and Confident Under Stress*, https://doi.org/10.1007/978-3-662-64440-9_2

2

In this chapter, I will describe what happens in our body when we are confronted with a stressor, that is a demand that threatens our physical and mental balance. This is a very complex event. This chapter is therefore quite extensive, in order to enable the interested reader to gain a good understanding of the respective connections. For those readers who are less interested in the biological side of the stress event, I recommend that they read the first two sections of this chapter and then continue with ▶ Sect. 2.8. This will give you a sufficient understanding of the most important biological factors of the stress event.

Physical signs of stress

So how does our body respond to the confrontation with a stressor? You, dear readers, have certainly noticed the typical physical signs of stress in yourself: The heart is pounding. Breathing becomes faster and shallower. The muscles, especially in the neck, shoulders, and back, tense up. We often begin to sweat. The mouth becomes dry. Often we feel a dull feeling in the stomach area, shaky hands, and knees, and above all this diffuse and at the same time penetrating feeling of inner restlessness and nervousness.

The stress response is the normal biological response to danger

The physical stress response encompasses a wide range of biological processes, all of which contribute to our physical activation and mobilization of energy. The physical stress response is a completely normal biological process. It was developed by nature during evolution as a program to ensure our own survival in dangerous situations. The physical activation brought about by the stress reaction does not—and this is important to emphasize from the very beginning—a priori and in any case represent a health hazard but is a normal response of the body to threats to the physical and mental balance as provided by nature. Under what circumstances and in what ways this intrinsically normal physical activation under stress can become a health risk will be discussed at the end of this chapter. But let us first take a closer look at what the physical stress reaction consists of in detail, what its purpose is and how it is set in motion.

2.1 The Body's Response to Stress: The General Adaptation Syndrome

General Adaptation Syndrome

The Austrian-Canadian physician and biochemist Hans Selye (1907–1982), who is now considered the father of modern stress research, was the first to systematically study the physical stress response. In extensive animal experiments and observations on humans, he discovered that organisms responded to very different stresses with always the same typical physical changes. No matter whether the animals were exposed to loud noise, extreme heat or cold, were deprived of food, had to endure uncontrollable electric shocks, or were kept in over-populated cages, in all cases they always showed the same characteristic physical responses, namely the stress reaction. Selye also called this **General Adaptation Syndrome (GAS).** With this, he wanted to express that the stress reaction is an unspecific, even general reaction of the organism to various kinds of stressors, which serves the physical adaptation of the organism to these stressors.

The stress response is a very comprehensive physical response to stress that affects all important organ systems and functions. The most important physical effects of acute activation of the biological stress program are shown in ◗ Fig. 2.1.

Stress affects all important organs

■ **Brain**

The blood circulation in the brain is increased, and the nerve tracts are activated. The brain is awake and focused. The sensory organs are directed outwards to be able to absorb and process new information from the environment at lightning speed. At the same time, access to memory content is made more difficult.

■ **Breathing**

The bronchi dilate and breathing become faster and shallow. Chest breathing dominates over diaphragmatic breathing. The emphasis of breathing is placed on inhalation, while exhala-

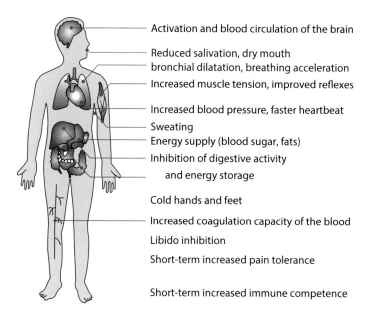

Activation and blood circulation of the brain

Reduced salivation, dry mouth
bronchial dilatation, breathing acceleration

Increased muscle tension, improved reflexes

Increased blood pressure, faster heartbeat

Sweating

Energy supply (blood sugar, fats)

Inhibition of digestive activity
and energy storage

Cold hands and feet

Increased coagulation capacity of the blood

Libido inhibition

Short-term increased pain tolerance

Short-term increased immune competence

◗ **Fig. 2.1** Physical reactions under stress

2

tion is less deep. This results in the body being better supplied with oxygen.

■ Cardiovascular

The heart is better supplied with blood and more efficient. It beats faster and stronger, so it can pump more volume of blood per unit of time into the veins. We often feel the heart pounding up to the neck. The blood pressure also rises. The blood vessels of the heart, the brain (redhead!), and the large working muscles continue to expand. At the same time, the blood vessels of the skin, the body periphery (cold hands and feet!), and the digestive tract constrict. This leads to a redistribution of the blood with the result of improved blood circulation and energy supply to the heart, brain, and muscles.

■ Musculature

The blood circulation of the skeletal muscles is improved, thus ensuring the supply of oxygen and energy in the form of fats for burning in the muscles. Muscle tension is increased, especially in the shoulder, neck, and back muscles. The shoulder girdle is often instinctively pulled up to protect the sensitive neck. The abdominal wall is rather tense to protect the intestines. The motor reflexes are improved, as is the reflex speed. All these changes serve to prepare the body for muscle work.

■ Metabolism

Sugar reserves from the liver are increasingly released into the blood and made available for consumption, especially for the brain. Fatty acids from the body's fat reserves are released into the blood for combustion in the muscles. At the same time, the digestive activity of the stomach and intestines is inhibited. This already begins with the reduced salivary flow, which is often clearly noticeable as a "dry mouth". Sometimes, acute stress can also lead to a strong urge to urinate and defecate and even to sudden diarrhoea. These reactions are by no means an expression of increased digestive activity; on the contrary, they indicate a severe loss of tone of the intestinal muscles and a "shutdown" of the digestive functions. In a way, the body gets rid of unnecessary ballast. Overall: The organism adjusts to a catabolic metabolic state, that is to energy consumption, while anabolic metabolic processes, that is those processes that serve to store energy, are slowed down.

■ Skin

Energy production generates heat which the body has to release to the outside to prevent possible overheating. This happens mainly through increased sweating, preferably on the hands, forehead, and armpits.

■ **Sexuality**

The sexual desire (the libido) is inhibited. The genital organs are also less supplied with blood. The release of male and female sex hormones is reduced. The male testicles produce fewer sperm, and the natural female cycle can be disturbed or, in extreme cases, completely interrupted. Overall, under acute stress, responsiveness to sexual stimuli is limited.

■ **Immune System**

Under acute stress, there is an increase in the natural killer cells in the blood. As a result, foreign bodies that have entered the bloodstream via open wounds or body orifices, for example, can be quickly recognized and rendered harmless. However, after only 30–60 min, the immune functions are throttled back in order to prevent an excessive immune reaction in the form of allergic reactions and to dampen inflammatory reactions.

■ **Pain**

The increased secretion of endogenous pain inhibitors, the endorphins, leads to a reduced sensitivity to pain and even to the so-called stress analgesia, that is an extensive insensitivity to painful stimuli. However, as the endorphin stores are limited, this pain-inhibiting effect only lasts for a short time. Longer lasting stress episodes therefore lead to reduced pain tolerance, that is an increased sensitivity to pain.

2.2 The Meaning of Physical Stress Response: Preparation for Fight or Flight

If we look at the different reactions that are set in motion in the body in response to stress, we can easily see the purpose of this biological program. Think of the prehistoric man in the distant past who encounters dangerous animals in his search for food, or of animals in the wild who face attacks from rival species. In such situations, there are basically two possibilities: Fight or flight. In both cases, this means intensive physical activity. And this is exactly what the stress reaction enables us to do. It prepares us in the shortest possible time and in the best possible way to counter an imminent danger with major motor action, with a **fight or flight reaction**. Those bodily functions that are necessary for the execution of such a physical coping reaction are stimulated (breathing, cardiovascular system, energy supply), while the more regenerative and reproductive bodily functions (digestion and energy storage, sexuality, reproduction, growth), which are less important for the short-term confrontation with an acute danger, are curbed.

Preparation for fight or flight

2

Survival advantage through a stress reaction

The development of the biological stress program in the course of evolution is almost a stroke of genius of nature. It gave an enormous survival advantage to the creatures that were equipped with this program. In contrast to living beings with rigid behavioural programmes (instincts) that failed in unforeseeable situations, the stress reaction as a non-specific activation programme enabled a flexible coping with the most varied, even new, dangerous situations. The activation of this program can also be useful for today's humans in all those situations where a quick physical reaction is required. However, it proves to be less functional in many of the particularly performance-related and socially demanding situations with which people today are confronted, in so far as the stress-related physical and emotional activation does not support a constructive coping with this demand, but often rather hinders it.

2.3 Stress Originates in the Brain

How is the stress reaction set in motion? Where and how is it triggered? And how are the described reactions of the various organ systems involved in the stress reaction controlled? We will deal with these questions in the following sections.

The complexity of the brain

The control centre for the stress reaction is the brain. The human brain is without doubt the most complex structure that nature has produced. If you take a closer look at the brain, you cannot help but be astonished. The complexity goes far beyond anything you can imagine. Even the number of elements involved is intimidating. The number of nerve cells is estimated at about 100 billion. Each nerve cell is connected to other nerve cells by up to 10,000 connecting points (synapses). The total number of synapses is in the trillions. A brain mass the size of a match head contains an estimated 1 billion synapses. It is important to note that the connections between the neurons (intracortical connections) strongly predominate those that come from outside the brain via the sensory organs, and those that go outside for motor functions. There are about 5 million intracortical connections per incoming or outgoing fibre. This fact makes it clear that the brain is not a simple stimulus-response apparatus but a highly complex information processor.

The brain as an information processor

Through the senses, we constantly absorb information from our environment. The sensory organs transform this information into biological signals and transmit them to the brain. The "input" flowing in via the sensory channels is combined and evaluated in the brain within fractions of a second to form an "inner picture". Depending on how this inner picture turns out, the brain then triggers corresponding responses. For this purpose, the brain uses electrical nerve impulses and chemical nerve messengers, the so-called neurotransmitters, to send corresponding commands, for example, to the muscles, and it initiates the production of endogenous messengers, the so-called hormones, which transmit messages that are understood by all important organs of the body.

In everyday life, this processing of signals takes place continuously and is usually not very spectacular, that it does not usually lead to stronger body reactions. Only when the evaluation of the incoming information has led to the conclusion that a dangerous or alarm situation exists, does the brain trigger massive physical reactions, precisely the stress reaction. This is a complex process in which the following three brain parts are essentially involved:

- **Brain Stem**

The brain stem is the oldest part of the brain in evolutionary terms. It is the part of the brain adjacent to the spinal cord, where all information coming from the body converges and is passed on to the higher brain centres. The brain stem is responsible for automated, involuntary life functions. Its structures control, among other things, heart rate, blood pressure, and respiration. It is sometimes referred to as the "reptilian brain" because it can only ever react. Of particular importance for the stress reaction is the so-called blue nucleus (Locus coeruleus), a small cell nucleus area in the transition from the brain to the spinal cord. Its nerve cells produce about three quarters of one of the most important neurotransmitters in the brain, namely norepinephrine (also called noradrenaline). As we will see below, norepinephrine plays a decisive role in triggering the stress reaction.

The brain stem

- **Limbic System**

This is an area of nerve cell networks grouped around the brain stem in the form of a belt, which establishes a connection between the cerebrum and older, lower brain regions via a variety of ascending and descending pathways. The limbic system includes the thalamus, the amygdala, and the hypothalamus. The thalamus is the first switch point for the processing of sensory information flowing in via the sensory channels. From here, the signals are transmitted to the cerebral cortex, but in the thalamus itself a first, still very rudimentary evaluation of the incoming information already takes place. Emotional experiences are deeply stored in the amygdala. It plays a central role in triggering emotions, especially fear, and plays a leading role in controlling the stress reaction. The hypothalamus is the control centre for the regulation of many

The limbic system

2

basic vegetative functions (body temperature, water balance, hunger, and thirst) and controls the balance of many hormones in the body. Due to its tasks, the limbic system can be called the "emotional brain". In a sense, it is our centre for emotional intelligence.

■ **Cerebral Cortex**

The cerebral cortex

The cerebral cortex represents the youngest part of the human brain in terms of developmental history. It is responsible for conscious perception and all cognitive processes and is in a sense the "thinking brain". The signals coming from the outside world via the five senses are assembled here to form an "inner picture" of the world. The current situation is evaluated by comparing it with stored memories of similar situations. Also, the cerebral cortex can anticipate, that is it can anticipate dangerous situations that have not yet occurred in the imagination by means of initial clues.

The brain triggers the stress reaction

When we are confronted with a new situation, the incoming information is processed in these three parts of the brain and passed between them, and a "decision" is made to trigger a stress reaction. The sensory information transmitted by the sensory cells first converges in the thalamus, the first switch point, and from there passed on to the cerebral cortex, where precise processing of the information takes place. For this purpose, the brain accesses stored memories of similar situations. It compares the current situation with these memories. Situations that evoke memories of situations in which bad experiences were made, which could not be overcome, in which one felt helpless, are considered dangerous. Personal experiences, especially unpleasant and fearful previous experiences, which are stored in the nerve cell networks of the brain, are thus of decisive importance for triggering an acute stress reaction.

Interaction of the three brain parts

If the cerebrum, based on a comparison with previous experiences, comes to the conclusion that there is currently a danger, it triggers the stress reaction. The amygdala in the limbic system takes over the leading role. Its activation causes strong feelings of anxiety and possibly also anger and rage and further physical stress reactions are set in motion.

2.4 If Stress Reactions Precede Thought...

Most people know the experience that in certain situations (e.g. in traffic or during an argument) violent physical (palpitations, sweating, muscle tension, etc.) and emotional (fear, anger, etc.) stress reactions are triggered so quickly, almost reflexively, that there is no time at all for cognitive considerations, assessments, and decisions. These are only made in a second step and only clarify afterwards whether the alarm reaction is justified at all.

Stress reaction as "short circuit"

Emotional and physical stress reactions precede conscious mental assessments and evaluations. Modern brain research has now discovered the neuroanatomical and physiological basis for this phenomenon. Already in the thalamus, the first processing stage of the incoming information, a first, still very imprecise picture of the situation is formed. If a danger signal is already recognized here, the thalamus can also directly—bypassing the cerebral cortex in a kind of "short circuit"—trigger a stress reaction. In this case, the information about the threatening dangerous situation goes from the thalamus directly to the amygdala, which then immediately triggers the stress reaction. This mechanism explains the experience that physical and emotional stress reactions in some situations (e.g. in traffic, during an argument) occur so quickly and quasi reflexively that there is no time at all for conscious reflection (◘ Fig. 2.2).

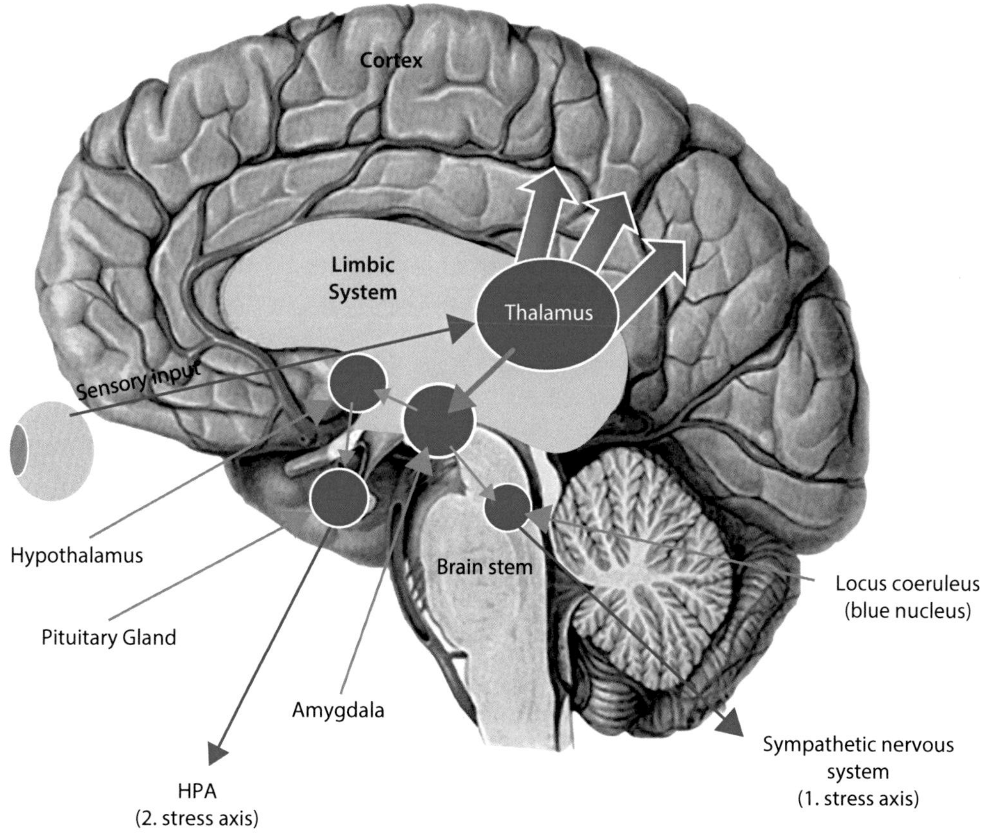

◘ **Fig. 2.2** Processing of stress stimuli in the brain (explanations in the text)

2

Life saver or false alarm

What comes from the thalamus is only a rough picture of the outside world, but it is transmitted very quickly. The amygdala thus learns of a potential danger just as quickly as the cerebral cortex: before you know what is actually going on, you already carry out the first involuntary protective reaction under emotional control. The cerebral cortex provides much sharper and more detailed images, but they need more time. In tricky situations, such a rapid short-circuit action can save lives under certain circumstances, but in other situations, it can also trigger physical and emotional stress reactions that, when looked at later, turn out to be inappropriate.

2.5 The Two Axes of Stress Response: Dry and Wet Communication Channels

If the brain comes to the conclusion that a threatening situation exists, it calls for a state of alarm. The nerve cells of the amygdala are activated. This gives the activation a strong emotional tone. We experience fear or anger. At the same time, the nerve cells of the amygdala begin to send out alarm signals by releasing large quantities of excitatory nerve messengers (glutamate) at their synapses. The amygdala nucleus thus alarms the stress centre in the brain stem, the "blue nucleus".

Sympathetic adrenal medulla axis

From here, from the "blue nucleus", the first immediate physical activation reaction is then triggered via the so-called sympathetic adrenal medulla axis: the nerve cells of the blue nucleus produce the neurotransmitter norepinephrine. This in turn activates the sympathetic nervous system, a nerve cord of the autonomic nervous system that runs along the spinal column and innervates all important organs and vessels. In fractions of a second, the nerve endings of the sympathetic nervous system in turn release norepinephrine, thereby stimulating respiration, pulse, and circulation.

Stress hormone adrenalin

Finally, the alarm message along the sympathetic nerve cord reaches the adrenal glands, small hat-like structures that sit on the kidneys and act as "hormone factories". The alarm signals transmitted by the sympathetic nervous system stimulate the medulla of the adrenal glands to release adrenaline commonly known as the stress hormone. Norepinephrine and adrenaline cause immediate activation of respiration, circulation, and energy supply. We are ready for fight or flight.

Hypothalamus–pituitary–adrenal cortex axis

If we succeed in escaping the danger or actively managing it, the stress programme is terminated. The "blue nucleus" stops sending alarm signals, the sympathetic activation decreases, the body calms down. The stress reaction comes to an end. The adrenaline in the blood is reduced; the body can recover.

If this is not the case, however, and the situation proves to be not so easily controlled, the activation of the amygdala and the "blue nucleus" is maintained. The nerve cells of the "blue nucleus" continue to release norepinephrine. This maintains the sympathetic activation. The amygdala continues to produce the excitatory messenger substance glutamate. This spreads via ascending nerve tracts also in higher brain regions. The activation of the cerebral cortex and the limbic system is intensified. This leads to an upswept and spreading excitation pattern, which eventually also affects specific nerve cell networks in the hypothalamus. The activation of these hypothalamic nerve cells in turn causes the stimulation of the second stress axis, the so-called **hypothalamic–pituitary–adrenal cortex axis (HPA axis)**. This consists of a whole cascade of coordinated hormonal reactions. In the hypothalamus, the superior control centre, the corticotropin-releasing factor (CRF) is released, a hormone that reaches the pituitary gland via a vascular system. There it stimulates the secretion of the adrenocorticotropic hormone (ACTH). This in turn enters the circulation and stimulates the release of cortisol in the adrenal cortex.

Cortisol is the second important stress hormone besides adrenaline. It makes a wide range of stress adjustments possible, ranging from increased provision of the energy-supplying blood sugar to fine-tuning of the immune system. Cortisol prepares the organism for a longer lasting confrontation with the stressful situation. To prevent the hormonal stress reaction from overreacting, the system has a feedback mechanism. The level of the cortisol in the blood is fed back to the superordinate switch points in the hypothalamus and the pituitary gland. A lot of cortisol in the blood inhibits the further release of the two releasing hormones CRH and ACTH. This is therefore a negative feedback mechanism that acts like a "stress brake" and causes the hormonal stress response to normally limit itself (◨ Fig. 2.3).

The activation of these two stress axes and the resulting release of the stress hormones adrenaline and cortisol represent, it should be emphasized again, completely normal biological processes and not per se a health risk. How this natural adaptation reaction can slip away in such a way that it leads to a health hazard and will be discussed at the end of this chapter.

Stress hormone cortisol

2

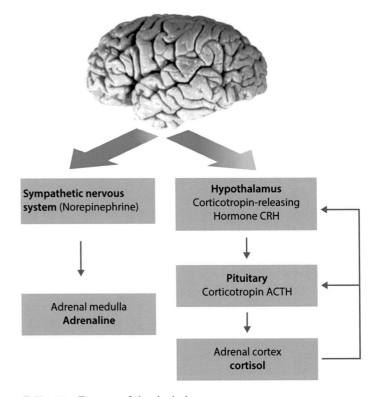

◨ **Fig. 2.3**   Two axes of the physical stress response

Conclusion

We can sum up here: When a situation is perceived as threat-ening, the sympathetic adrenal medulla axis is initially acti-vated and the first stress hormone, adrenaline, is released. The signal is transmitted "dry" via electrical impulses along the nerve tracts and is very fast. The function of this axis is the acute activation of the heart, circulation, and respiration. Figuratively speaking, it corresponds to a "call to arms". If the dangerous situation persists, that is if the perceived danger cannot be brought under control despite all efforts, the second axis, the hypothalamic–pituitary–adrenal cortex axis, is also activated and the second stress hormone, cor-tisol, is released. The signal transmission here is "wet" in a sense, as it takes place via hormone releases into the blood. It takes place much more slowly than in the nervous system. Metaphorically speaking, the function of this axis consists in organizing replenishment in the form of energy supply. In this way, the organism prepares itself for a longer lasting confron-tation with the dangerous situation.

2.6 Stress Shapes the Brain

In the previous presentation, we have considered the brain exclusively as the starting point of the stress reaction with its manifold physical effects. However, the brain is also the target organ of the stress reaction. Both noradrenaline and cortisol have far-reaching effects on the functioning of the brain. Of particular interest, here are the effects of stress hormones on the neuronal circuits in the brain.

Stress hormones influence the brain

Fundamental to the understanding of these effects is the central insight of modern neurobiological brain research into **neuronal plasticity.** This refers to the brain's basic ability to change the connections between nerve cells depending on their use, thus rebuilding its own fine structure. Nerve cell connections that are frequently used in the context of perceptions or activities are stabilized or reinforced. Conversely, connections between nerve cells that are activated very little are inhibited and can be lost altogether. Neurobiologists have summed up this finding with the striking formula **"Use it or lose it"**.

Neuronal plasticity

For example, in violin and guitar players, the nerve cell clusters in the sensorimotor cortex that control the movements of the second to the fifth finger are particularly pronounced compared to non-musicians. When playing stops, these neuronal structures regress. Incidentally, similar findings were also found in young people who frequently sent text messages compared to older people. To a certain extent, the use-dependent plasticity of the brain provides the neurobiological basis for learning.

The realization that our brain virtually forms itself depending on its use was groundbreaking and has thoroughly revised the earlier idea that we are born with a "finished" brain and that from birth onwards there is only an unstoppable breakdown of nerve cells. In the meantime, the biological processes that enable the formation of nerve cell connections have also been extensively researched. Nerve cells that are activated do something for their self-preservation. When activated, they also produce certain proteins that serve as nerve growth factors. These proteins promote the expulsion of axons that bring the nerve cells into contact with each other, and strengthen the synapses, the actual contact points. It is basically the same as with muscles. The muscles that we use and train regularly grow and become stronger and muscles that are not used lose mass and become flabbier.

Nerve growth factors

2

> What does all this have to do with stress? What is decisive here is the fact that stress, or more precisely the neurotransmitters and hormones released during stress, influences the production and release of precisely these nerve growth factors.

Noradrenaline breaks down neuronal circuits

Noradrenaline, which is released in the brain as part of the acute stress reaction, promotes the release of neurotrophic factors (growth-promoting substances for nerve cells), which in turn lead to increased growth of axons and the formation of synapses. The repeated noradrenergic activation during short-term controllable stress leads to a better development, a better pathway, and more effective functioning of all the circuits that are used in our brain to cope with a demand.

Cortisol inhibits neuronal circuits

Cortisol, which is released during a prolonged stress episode and circulates in the blood, also reaches the brain without any problems. There, depending on the dose and duration of exposure, it causes lasting changes in the nerve cells that are opposite to those of noradrenaline. The cortisol release associated with long-term uncontrollable stress leads to the suppression of the synthesis and release of neurotrophic factors. As a result, existing neuronal circuits are inhibited and destabilized.

These effects of stress hormones on the neuronal circuits in the brain are also biologically useful. As long as we are confronted with a danger, which we are able to control by means of the acute stress reaction, those nerve cell networks in the brain are stabilized under the influence of norepinephrine, in which the behaviours are stored, with which we have managed to cope with the danger. The brain memorizes the behaviour pattern with which the situation was successfully mastered. It builds up the corresponding neural circuits so that it can react even faster in a similar situation in the future.

If, however, the situation proves to be less easy to control and longer stress reactions occur, the brain now begins, under the influence of cortisol, to inhibit and break down the nerve cell networks that store the behaviours that have proven to be unsuitable for eliminating the danger. In a sense, the brain deletes these patterns of behaviour, thereby creating the conditions for us to develop and try out new behaviours.

> Stress thus proves to be an important catalyst for learning processes.

Memory disorders—a possible consequence of permanent stress

Stress hormones promote adaptation by facilitating the formation of experiences as well as the processing of novel stimuli. This applies as long as short-term stress reactions are involved. In the case of long-lasting chronic stress reactions, there can be massive damaging effects on the neuronal structures in certain brain regions. The American stress researcher Robert Sapolsky from Stanford University, for example, found in apes that were permanently stressed by conflicts and stressful relationships within their horde, a shrinkage of a brain structure called the hippocampus, which plays a particular important role in memory. In the meantime, research findings show that this is not only true for great apes but also for humans.

2.7 Stress Reactions Are Individual

So far ,we have learned about the most important physical stress reactions and the complex ways in which they are controlled. However, the biological stress programme does not always run in the same stereotypical way for all people in all stress situations. Some people primarily react with the digestive system when under stress and above all sense the queasy feeling in the stomach. Others focus on activating the cardiovascular system, the heart beats, the blood shoots into the head. And still others respond primarily by tensing the muscles. Knowing your own individual stress reaction patterns and perceiving them as sensitively and early as possible is a prerequisite for successful stress management. If we pay attention to our personal physical stress signals (instead of ignoring them for as long as possible, which unfortunately often happens), then we have a kind of early warning system at our disposal that can help us to take timely countermeasures. It is therefore important to train the perception of the stress signals of your own body (▶ Box 2.1).

Individual stress signals as an early warning system

> **Box 2.1: Self-monitoring: What Are My Personal Physical Stress Signals?**
> In the coming days, please pay close attention to the first signs that your body is signaling to you that it is stressed. Where and how is the tension most likely to be felt in your body? These early warning signals are very diverse and vary from person to person. For many people, it is mainly muscular tension, especially in the neck and shoulder muscles. Under stress, they retract the head and raise the shoulders as if they were trying to form a shell. Others bite their teeth together and react with a strong tension of the jaw muscles or teeth grinding. Still others tense the forehead, causing deep wrinkles on the forehead, and they feel the pressure mainly in the head and around the eyes. A frequent stress signal is also a dull feeling in the stomach area, sometimes slight diarrhoea or an increased urge to urinate. And again and again, it hap-

2

pens that stress signals are expressed by individual physical weak points, for example, old scars, gingivitis, haemorrhoids, or herpes blisters, which become unpleasantly noticeable. If we know and pay attention to the stress signals of our body, we have the chance to take countermeasures in time before more serious health problems occur.

2.8 The Shaping of the Stress Response Through Early Experiences

Early childhood experiences shape the biological stress system

The sensitivity of the stress axes also varies from individual to individual. Numerous scientific studies in the stress laboratory confirm the everyday observation that people who find themselves in the same "objective" stress situation differ significantly from one another in terms of the strength of the physical stress reactions that occur. The differences are particularly clear with regard to the activation of the second stress axis, the HPA axis, and the associated release of CRF, ACTH, and finally cortisol (see above). The initially obvious assumption that these differences in the individual stress response are genetically determined and inherited could not be confirmed by studies in twins. Instead, it is now assumed that the biological stress system is essentially shaped by early childhood experiences.

Maternal care as a protective factor

A decisive role in this is played by the amount of affection one has experienced in early childhood. In various studies on animals, the Canadian stress researcher Michael Meaney, for example, was able to show that the intensity of maternal attention in the first period after birth plays a decisive role in how intensively stress hormones are released later in the adult animals under stressful conditions. Lovingly mothered young animals showed a significantly lower release of stress hormones than animals that had received little attention as newborns. The attention given in early childhood acts as a kind of protective mantle into adulthood.

Separation from the mother as stressor

The separation from the mother in the period after birth is a very strong stressor for young animals and leads to a lasting sensitization of the biological stress system. Stress researchers at Stanford University found in apes that were separated from their mother early after birth, in a later study after 3 years, strongly increased reactions of the second stress axis in a stressful situation. More recent research shows that this is probably due to the fact that the young animals do not develop a functioning "stress brake" (see above).

Scientific observations in humans also confirm this: A secure bond between the infant and its mother (or another caregiver) provides an effective protective shield against stress into adulthood. And vice versa: Insecure bonds in early childhood lead to increased and prolonged activity of the second stress axis in stressful situations in adult life, measurable, for example, by increased cortisol concentrations in the blood.

One reason for an insecure binding may be that the mother (or another primary caregiver) herself—for whatever reason—is too stressed. She is then too preoccupied with her own feelings of stress, fear, insecurity, or helplessness and cannot take sufficient and emphatic care of the child. This is also shown by the results of studies conducted by the research group of the American neurobiologist Charles Nemeroff at the Primate Centre in New York. Monkey mothers were put under stress in different ways after birth. The result was that the young animals of stressed mothers reacted later, when they themselves were put under stress, with a stronger biological stress response than young animals of "relaxed" mothers. This shows how a certain susceptibility to stress is less inherited biologically than is passed on more socially.

Protection through secure binding

If the mother is too stressed…

> **Conclusion**
>
> In summary, we can state that past experiences influence the current stress experience in later life in two ways. Firstly, past experiences of coping with difficult situations stored in the brain are the yardstick against which the assessment of a current requirement is made. Secondly, early stress and attachment experiences leave an imprint in the biological stress system, alter the sensitivity of the stress axes and thus shape the intensity of the stress experience in adulthood.

2.9 Does Stress Make You Ill? How Stress Endangers Health

To reiterate: the physical activation triggered by a stressor is not in itself harmful to health. On the contrary: "Stress is the spice of life", as Hans Selye, the pioneer of stress research, once put it. Which means that short-term activation, which is constantly alternating with phases of relaxation, is a significant positive characteristic of the living. This can be seen not only in the natural sleep-wake rhythm, but also in such fundamental physiological processes as the activity of the heart muscle with its constant alternation of systole and diastole, as well as in the rhythmic alternation of inhalation and exhala-

Alternation of tension and relaxation—a basic principle of life

2

tion during the breathing process. Phasic activation as an expression of vitality is subjectively experienced as pleasant and full of relish and has a performance-enhancing and motivating effect. Selye speaks in this case of "eustress", which he distinguishes from "distress", which is dangerous to health.

A risk to physical health due to stress reactions does not arise from the mere fact of short-term physical activation. The following four main aspects are important for the adverse health effects of physical stress reactions:

■ **Energy Not Consumed**

Provided energy is not consumed

The physical stress reactions described above are a very old reaction pattern in terms of developmental history, by means of which the organism is optimally prepared to meet dangerous situations by fighting or fleeing. The preparation for attack and flight was originally biologically expedient for coping with exactly the demands to which animals and also prehistoric man were primarily exposed. The defence of one's own territory against enemy species, the exploitation of food, rank fights, the defence against wild animals—all these demands required physical activity, which prepared the stress programme in an optimal way. By coping with the demands in a physical way, by fighting or fleeing, the stress reaction was brought to its natural end. The sugar and fat reserves provided were used up. After successful coping, the organism could come to rest and recover. In coping with many stressful situations of modern man, however, this reaction pattern has lost its immediate adaptability, as physical attacks or escape attempts are rarely an appropriate response to the stressors of modern life. Thus, the energy provided is not consumed. Fat, sugar, and clumping blood platelets block the bloodstream. This can lead to vasoconstriction (arteriosclerosis) and finally to complete vascular occlusion (infarction) in the heart, lungs, or brain.

The consequence that can be drawn from this for the prevention of stress-related health risks is obvious: we must ensure regular physical activity in order to actually consume the energy provided in the stress reaction. Sport and physical activity as an important part of any successful anti-stress strategy will be discussed in more detail in ▶ Sect. 8.4.

■ **Chronic Stress**

No time for relaxation

The stress response has evolved over the course of evolution as a program for dealing with hazards that are of relatively short duration. However, many of the stressors that are important to modern man, for example, in the interpersonal or professional sphere, are characterized by the fact that they persist over a long period of time, often for years, or that they recur again and again. Thus, the necessary time for recovery and relaxation is often missing. The organism is constantly kept in a state of increased activation. Finally, if the strain is sustained for too long, the organism's ability to adapt breaks down. In this so-called stage of exhaustion, a wide range of functional symptoms can occur, including serious organ diseases.

The tension becomes chronic

In addition, if the increased resistance level is maintained over a long period of time, the organism gradually loses its natural ability to self-regulate. This means that it is no longer possible to return to a normal resting level even in phases when there is no acute stress. The walls of the blood vessels lose their elasticity, and the vessels can no longer dilate, with the result that blood pressure remains chronically elevated. Tense, painful muscles are difficult to loosen and may even trigger further muscular tension reactions by reflection, thus creating a vicious circle through which the tension is continuously maintained. Recovery—even during sleep—occurs more and more slowly, if at all. The hypothalamus–pituitary–adrenal cortex axis remains permanently activated. The mechanism of negative feedback, the so-called stress brake, which causes self-limitation of cortisol release, is suspended. Chronically elevated cortisol levels are found in the blood. These have a complex effect on various physiological functions.

For example, on insulin production in the pancreas: cortisol reduces the effect of insulin, which normally promotes the absorption of sugar into the body's cells. As a result, more sugar remains in the blood and can enter the brain as an energy carrier, whose cells do not need insulin to absorb sugar. In the pancreas, the reduced insulin effect caused by cortisol is registered, "interpreted" as a relative insulin deficiency and answered with increased insulin production. In the longer term, the production capacity for insulin in the islet cells of the pancreas is exhausted. This results in an actual insulin deficiency, which increases blood sugar levels and thus the risk of diabetes.

Example diabetes

Chronified stress reactions due to long-lasting or recurring stress, that is permanent stress, represent an enormous health risk. The consequence of this for prevention is obvious: we must ensure regular compensation, regular phases of relaxation and regeneration, also and especially in phases of longer lasting high demands. How this can be achieved will be dealt with intensively in ► Chap. 8.

■ **Weakened Immune System**

Scientific studies show that under stress the body's own defences of the immune system can be sustainably influenced. With short-term acute stress, the immune system is first stimu-

The immune system is weakened

2

lated. This increases the number of natural killer cells in the blood. In a sense, these form the organism's first line of defence against foreign bodies that enter the organism from outside, for example, via open wounds. Such foreign bodies can then be recognised more quickly and fought more effectively. These immunostimulatory effects occur during the activation of the first stress axis, the sympathetic adrenal medulla axis, in the acute stress phase. If the stress continues, the activation of the second stress axis, the hypothalamus–pituitary–adrenal cortex axis, leads to an increased release of the stress hormone cortisol. This hormone, when released over a longer period of time under constant stress, causes a sustained weakening of our immune system. This is accompanied by a generally increased susceptibility to infectious diseases, for example, colds and herpes virus infections.

If you can't get "really sick"...

For example, cold viruses (so-called rhinoviruses) lead to an actual cold more often in stressed people than in unstressed people. If an infection has then occurred, chronically elevated cortisol levels additionally hinder their effective control; because cortisol suppresses fever reactions, inflammatory reactions, and other important defence reactions of the body. Colds, herpes infections, or inflamed wounds then drag on without healing properly. You may be sick somehow, but you cannot become "really sick". Many people know this from their everyday experience: they have picked up an infection, but it remains largely silent during the week under the pressure of professional demands. You may feel slight symptoms, a scratching in the throat, tingling in the nose or slight shivering. But often the infection and the body's own defensive reactions, for example, in the form of fever, really come to the fore not until the weekend, when the stress and thus the influence of the cortisol subsides.

Weakened immune competence and chronic diseases

The weakening of the immune system caused by chronically elevated cortisol levels can also have an unfavourable effect on the course of such diseases, which themselves have nothing to do with stress. This is particularly true for those often chronic diseases in which inflammatory processes in the body or the immune system itself play a role. These include diseases such as multiple sclerosis, rheumatoid arthritis, skin diseases such as psoriasis, but also various tumour diseases.

Chronically elevated cortisol levels caused by constant stress impair the body's ability to deal with these diseases. In order to prevent stress-related weakening of the immune system, it is important that we strengthen the immune system through a health-conscious lifestyle, especially through healthy eating and sufficient exercise in the fresh air, and that we give the immune system the space to work. Since the immune system does much of its work while we sleep, this means in particular that we must ensure that we get sufficient and restful sleep (see also ▶ Sect. 8.1).

■ **Health Risk Behaviour**

Stress-related health risks often result from the fact that many people under stress increasingly resort to behaviour that is harmful to their health. They smoke more than usual, drink alcohol excessively or uncontrollably, eat irregularly, and often eat unhealthily or neglect exercise. In this way, they try to get a grip on the demands and, even more so, the feelings of stress that arise. However, these are unsuitable coping attempts in the long term. On the one hand, these behaviours directly increase the risk of numerous diseases. And on the other hand, they reduce the resilience towards stress in the long term and thus contribute to a more rapid exhaustion of the resistance forces.

Smoking and alcohol to calm down

■ **Chronic Stress and Physical Illness**

In view of the diverse effects of the stress response on practically all important organ systems, it is not surprising that the possible harmful effects of chronic stress reactions are also extremely diverse, and that stress can play a role in a wide range of diseases.

Possible consequences of chronic stress

■ **Brain**

Under permanent stress, the performance of the brain decreases. Especially memory, concentration and creativity are affected. The stress hormones also cause changes in the biochemistry of the brain, which in the long term can lead to depression.

■ **Cardiovascular**

The blood pressure remains elevated in the long term. This puts a strain on the heart muscle. Often the pulse is also elevated. The walls of the arteries are overloaded. This promotes inflammatory processes in the vessel wall with the development of calcifications (arteriosclerosis). Late consequences can be heart attack and stroke.

■ **Musculature**

Persistent tension of the muscles can lead to headache and neck and back pain.

■ **Metabolism**

Constant stress favours the development of diabetes. The increased release of fatty acids also leads to an unfavourable increase in the blood fat level. This promotes the deposition of fats in the arterial wall. The vessels constrict over time. High

2

blood pressure can be the result or even stroke or heart attack if a vein in the brain or heart is completely blocked by the deposition.

■ **Digestive Activity**
The body's own regulation is influenced in the long term, stomach ulcers and digestive problems increase.

■ **Sexuality**
Constant stress reduces sexual desire. It can lead to cycle disorders in women as well as impotence and disturbances in sperm maturation in men.

■ **Sensory Organs**
Under stress, the intraocular pressure can increase and promote the development of glaucoma. A frequent consequence of stress is damage to the inner ear, with sudden hearing loss and continuous whistling sounds (tinnitus).

■ **Immune System**
Constant stress weakens the immune system. Constant colds, flu, and bronchitis can be the result.
◘ Table 2.1 provides an—albeit not complete—overview of such diseases for the development and course of which also long-term consequences of chronic stress must be considered.

◘ **Table 2.1**   Chronic stress and physical illness

Long-term consequences	
Brain	– Restriction of cognitive performance and memory functions – Cerebral infarction
Sensory organs: eye, ear	– Increased intraocular pressure – Noises in the ear, tinnitus, sudden deafness
Cardiovascular	– High blood pressure – Arteriosclerosis – Coronary heart disease – Heart attack
Musculature	– Headache, backache – Soft tissue rheumatism
Digestive organs	– Digestive disorders – Gastrointestinal ulcers
Metabolism	– Increased blood sugar level/diabetes – Increased cholesterol level

☐ **Table 2.1** (continued)	
Long-term consequences	
Immune system	– Reduced immunocompetence in the face of infectious diseases, frequent infections – Unfavourable course of tumour diseases, multiple sclerosis, rheumatoid arthritis, among others
Pain	– Reduced pain tolerance – Increased pain experience
Sexuality	– Libido loss – Cycle disorders in women – Impotence – Disorders of semen maturation, infertility

Note: The table lists the most common physical illnesses that can be caused or influenced in their course by chronic stress. However, this does not mean that the respective illness is always and exclusively due to stress

■ **Chronic Stress and Mental Health**

Chronic stress not only has harmful effects on physical health but also causes disturbances in mental well-being and mental health. These emotional disorders often develop before the physical disorders. However, affected persons usually only go to the doctor when physical symptoms or diseases have also occurred. The doctor diagnoses and treats these physical disorders, but the associated chronic stress and mental disorders often remain undetected and correspondingly untreated.

Stress and mental disorders

There is now particularly good evidence of a connection between the occurrence of depressive disorders and overactivity of the second stress axis, the HPA axis. Many (but not all) depressive people, like people who are permanently stressed, have chronically elevated cortisol levels in their blood. These are mainly due to an overproduction of the corticotropin-releasing factor (CRF), which in turn is caused by a defect in the hypothalamus or a superior authority. The stress axis is therefore no longer fully subject to the mechanisms that normally downregulate it ("stress brake") and is therefore chronically activated. Based on these scientifically sufficiently proven correlations, the assumption is justified that many depressions (but not all) are a consequence of permanent stress. The Mainz psychiatrist and depression researcher Prof. Benkert speaks here quite explicitly of the widespread disease "stress depression", which affects up to 20% of the population and which—according to a study by the World Health Organization (WHO)—will be the most common disease worldwide in 2020, alongside cardiovascular diseases.

Widespread disease "stress depression"

2

2.10 Total Exhaustion: The Burnout Syndrome

Many people suffer from burnout

The term "burnout" (= "being burnt out") refers to a persistent and severe state of exhaustion as a result of a chronic stress reaction with both physical and mental symptoms. Those affected feel exhausted and empty, they feel that their work is meaningless and useless and they withdraw from other people. The first descriptions came from interaction-intensive fields of work, especially in helping professions with social workers, nurses, doctors, and teachers. Burnout was understood here in a narrow sense as exhaustion due to emotional stress caused by helping without adequate reward. In the meantime, burnout symptoms have been shown in members of many other professions, for example, police officers, managers, flight attendants and call centre staff, journalists, IT specialists (especially in start-up companies), architects, and top athletes. Burnout is also not limited to burdens associated with gainful employment. Rather, burnout processes can also result from long-term burdens from family-, care- and housework as well as voluntary work.

Burnout is not a clearly defined clinical picture, nor does it represent an independent psychiatric diagnosis. There is a wide range of symptomatic overlap, especially with depressive disorders and psychosomatic disorders. When patients go to the doctor—which is usually postponed again and again—it is usually because of the physical disorders, which are then diagnosed and treated symptomatically. The underlying burnout often remains undetected.

Recovery no longer successful

Metaphorically speaking, it is a long-lasting energy release with little effect and little energy replenishment, at least in later phases. The battery is empty and can no longer be charged. This is similar to the situation when a car battery is no longer recharged by the alternator, but still has to deliver maximum power. And this is also the difference to normal, "righteous" fatigue after a major effort. Burnout is characterized by a loss of the natural ability to regenerate. One cannot recover.

Burnout as a creeping process

Burnout does not happen from one day to the next, but it is a slow, creeping **process of burning out.** The development often begins with a longer phase of increased demands and strong commitment. Gradually, the first signs of diminishing performance creep in. Concentration decreases, errors increase, which then require additional "follow-up" work. Tiredness and feelings of weakness unknown up to now appear, sleep often becomes worse, and pain of all kinds also occurs more frequently. Those affected do not react to these first signs of beginning exhaustion by taking time out to recover and recharge their batteries. On the contrary: as they see no possibility to change their situation, they increase their commitment and try to compensate for the loss of performance by more commitment and even more work. If their own recovery needs are perceived at all, they (and their relatives) always put themselves off until "better times". There is an ever-increasing withdrawal from private contacts and from leisure activities. Perseverance is experienced as the only option; all available energy is concentrated on work. A vicious circle develops: one works longer but more and more ineffectively, which is why one has to work even longer. One feels more and more exhausted and is at the same time hyperactive in exhaustion. In this situation, those affected often resort more often to medication (stimulants, sleeping pills, painkillers) in order to combat loss of performance and symptoms of exhaustion. The further development towards complete exhaustion is already in sight. One affected person once described her path to burnout as follows: "For too long I have done too much for too many others with too little consideration for myself".

A fully developed burnout syndrome manifests itself in the physical, mental, emotional, and also in the social area. The most important **symptoms** are listed in the ► Box 2.2.

The **therapy** of a fully developed burnout syndrome is complex and time-consuming. It includes intensive psychotherapy to work on the underlying personal factors that have contributed to the burnout, physical therapy measures to treat the physical exhaustion symptoms and to restore the ability to regenerate as well as (psycho-)pharmacological treatment if necessary. Often an in-patient therapy in a clinic specialized in the treatment of burnout is necessary and advisable.

Therapy of the Burnout Syndrome

Box 2.2: The Most Important Symptoms of the Burnout Syndrome
— **Physical exhaustion**
  – Lack of energy, chronic fatigue, feelings of weakness,
  – Insomnia,
  – Weakened immune system (frequent infections),
  – Psychosomatic symptoms (headache, backache, gastrointestinal complaints, cardiovascular disorders),
  – Reduced libido, sexual dysfunction.

These physical exhaustion symptoms are often combated by increased consumption of alcohol and cigarettes as well as by taking painkillers, sleeping pills, sedatives, or stimulants.

2

- **Emotional exhaustion**
  - Surfeit: Everything is too much.
  - Despondency, hopelessness.
  - Feeling of inner emptiness, of being emotionally dead.
  - These can alternate with irritability, anger, blame.
- **Mental exhaustion**
  - Reduction of cognitive performance, lack of concentration, forgetfulness.
  - Loss of creativity.
  - Negative attitude towards oneself, work, life in general.
  - Cynicism.
  - Thoughts of futility.
- **Social exhaustion**
  - Loss of interest in others, social withdrawal (not only professionally but also privately).
  - Feelings of being sucked out by others, other people, are only experienced as "annoying" and as a further burden.
  - Loss of empathy (lack of understanding for others, not being able or willing to listen).
  - Depersonalization ("dehumanization"): other people (e.g. clients, patients, customers, colleagues) are depersonalized, treated only as cases or numbers.

2.11   Checklist: Warning Signs for Stress

Give up denial

In order to prevent this from happening in the first place, it is crucial to notice and observe the first symptoms of exhaustion as early as possible. However, this is often exactly where the problem lies. It is always amazing how long many people drag themselves along burnt out and try to avoid a (self-)critical examination of their own situation. This requires courage and the abandonment of denial, of not wanting to know and of trivialization. The courage to face one's own situation critically is, however, usually rewarded with the release of new energy, even a real liberation. Energy that was needed until then to maintain denial, to look away, to persist in the "ever-widening" and that can now be invested in changing one's own life situation.

Encourage self-exploration

◘ Figure 2.4 contains a checklist of frequent warning signals at physical, emotional, mental, and behavioural levels. Please use this list for an honest and open reflection of your current health condition.

Checklist: Warning signals for stress				

The following points can be signs of overstraining. Which of these do you have noticed about yourself in the last week?

	strong	moderate	hardly/ not at all	Points
Physical warning signals				
Heartbeats/heartstitches	2	1	0	
Tightness in the chest	2	1	0	
Breathing difficulties	2	1	0	
Insomnia	2	1	0	
Chronic fatigue	2	1	0	
Digestive disorders	2	1	0	
stomach pain	2	1	0	
Loss of appetite	2	1	0	
Sexual dysfunction	2	1	0	
Muscle Tensions	2	1	0	
Headaches	2	1	0	
Back pain	2	1	0	
Cold hands/feet	2	1	0	
Strong sweating	2	1	0	
Emotional warning signals				
Nervousness, inner restlessness	2	1	0	
Irritability, feelings of anger	2	1	0	
Feelings of fear, fear of failure	2	1	0	
Dissatisfaction/imbalance	2	1	0	
Listlessness (also sexual)	2	1	0	
Inner emptiness, "being burned out"	2	1	0	
Cognitive warning signals				
Constantly circling thoughts/rumination	2	1	0	
Concentration disorders	2	1	0	
Emptiness in the head ("black out")	2	1	0	
Daydreams	2	1	0	
Nightmares	2	1	0	
Loss of performance/frequent mistakes	2	1	0	

◘ **Fig. 2.4** Checklist: Warning signals for stress

2

	strong	moderate	hardly/ not at all	Points
Warning signals in behavior				
Aggressive behaviour towards others, "going off the deep end"	2	1	0	
finger drums, feet scratching, trembling, teeth crunch	2	1	0	
Speak fast or stutter	2	1	0	
Interrupting others, not being able to listen	2	1	0	
Eat irregularly	2	1	0	
consumption of alcohol (or medication) to calm down	2	1	0	
Let private contacts "grind"	2	1	0	
More smoking than desired	2	1	0	
Less sport and exercise than desired	2	1	0	
Total score				_____

Rating:

0-10 points

You can be happy about your relatively good health stability. A relaxation training will mainly have a preventive effect on you.

11-20 points

The chain reactions of physical and mental stress reactions are already taking place in your body. You should start as soon as possible to expand your stress management skills.

21 and more points

They are already deep in the vicious circle of tension, emotional stress and health problems. You should definitely do something about your stress and for more serenity, peace and efficiency.

◘ **Fig. 2.4**   (continued)

What Stresses Us: Stressors in Work and Everyday Life

Contents

© Springer-Verlag GmbH Germany, part of Springer Nature 2022
G. Kaluza, *Calm and Confident Under Stress*, https://doi.org/10.1007/978-3-662-64440-9_3

3

In this chapter, we will look in detail at the factors that trigger the biological stress programme, i.e. the stressors. We will look at the nature of the demands that primarily cause us stress today and what their characteristics are. We will also look at societal changes in the world of work and beyond, and what consequences these have for many people's experience of stress.

3.1 Requirements Promote Development

Every day, we successfully cope with a multitude of demands that we face in our professional and private lives. Training and experience have allowed us to develop routines that help us to cope with most everyday demands without stress. However, time and again we find ourselves in situations that confront us with demands and tasks that challenge or exceed the routines we have developed up to that point. Situations in which we are unsure of what to do and have to make an effort to find new ways. Situations that threaten our physical and mental equilibrium, that threaten the achievement of significant goals or the fulfillment of important motives and needs. In short, situations in which we get under stress.

Requirements as growth incentives

These situations are an important part of life. We need them in order to develop further. If we never expose ourselves to demands that we are not sure we can cope with, if we only ever confront ourselves with those demands that we know we can cope with on the basis of previous experience, then we would be stepping on the spot and would no longer develop further. Stressors, when properly "dosed", always represent growth stimuli. By dealing with them, we can develop new abilities, improve our skills, gain new insights, in short:

> ❯ Stressors represent opportunities or prompts for learning, they enable development.

Boredom in the land of milk and honey

A life entirely without stressors is, therefore, neither conceivable nor desirable. Rigidity in routine, boredom, stagnation, and ultimately physical and mental decay would be the consequences. The land of milk and honey comes from a horror fairy tale. Imagine a life without any demands: South Seas paradise, palm trees on the beach, hammock, no deadlines, no chores, no obligations, all-inclusive service—and forever. How long could you enjoy rocking in the hammock without becoming endlessly bored, without experiencing yourself as pointless or superfluous?

It is a misunderstanding that I occasionally encounter to think that the topic of "stress management" is about propagating a life that is as low in demands as possible, a life in a hammock, at an energetic zero line, so to speak. No, that is not what it is about, but rather a lively balance between phases of confrontation with demands, commitment, and engagement on the one hand, and phases of distancing, relaxation, and recuperation on the other. For the stimulation, development-promoting effect of stressors, their dose, that is their frequency, duration, and intensity, is of decisive importance. It is like physical training. Here, too, the intensity of the individual training sessions and the intervals at which they take place are crucial to achieving progress in training. Every sports trainer today knows that sufficient regeneration phases are an important part of the training itself, otherwise there is a danger of overtraining with a drop in performance.

It is the dose that counts

3.2 In the Foreground Today: Performance and Relationship Stress

While the biological stress program has remained unchanged over the millennia, this is not at all true for the factors that activate this program, that is, for the stressors. For prehistoric man, defending one's own territory against hostile conspecifics, capturing food, fighting for rank, and fending off wild animals were important stressors that threatened the physical balance. Today, we have to deal with completely different stressors that threaten not so much our physical equilibrium as our mental equilibrium (► Box 3.1).

> **Box 3.1: To Think Ahead: Modern Stressors—Which of These Do You Experience?**
> - Time stress: deadline pressure, hectic not only at work but also in private life.
> - Traffic stress: long drives to work, traffic jams, delays.
> - Information stress: flooding with or too little information.
> - Online stress: constant accessibility through smartphones, etc.
> - Density stress: overcrowding and confinement, for example, in buses and trains, on streets, in doctors' surgeries, lecture halls, and shops, at the same time isolation and anonymity in the masses.
> - Stress due to uncertainty and worries about the future.

3

Performance stressors

Time pressure

Stressors often arise in the area of performance, that is in the **fulfilment of tasks** in work, family, and household, when (too) many or too demanding everyday and professional requirements are (or have to be) met.

Surveys regularly show that the hit list of stressors is headed by time pressure. People have to or want to complete too many tasks in the time available. Depending on the target group, 50% to more than 80% of the people surveyed complain about "too little time". As a constantly present background stressor, time pressure determines professional and private everyday life. The causes are not always and exclusively to be found in the external demands, often personal attitudes and behaviours as well as an unfavourable time planning, contribute to the fact that time pressure arises. Are you one of the many people whose daily life is characterized by hectic and a chronic lack of time? If so, then take a moment to examine the following list (▶ Box 3.2) to find out which external and internal reasons are decisive for chronic time stress in your life.

Box 3.2: To Think Further: No Time?
Many factors contribute to the "no time" syndrome that is so prevalent today. Please take a self-critical look at the following list of reasons for chronic lack of time in your life.
 ▬ **External factors ("time eaters")**
  – Too many tasks
  – Phone
  – Constant interruptions
  – Too many, too long, badly prepared meetings
  – Lack of or incorrect information leading to delays
  – Unclear or constantly changing tasks
  – Superfluous paperwork, spam mails
  – Traffic jam
  – Long distances, long travel times
  – Queuing in the canteen
  – Unpunctual customers, clients
  – Unreliable employees or colleagues
  – Other: …
 ▬ **Own attitudes and behaviour**
  – Difficulty in setting priorities
  – Want to make things too perfect
  – Put off making decisions
  – Try to do everything at once
  – Put off unpleasant things
  – Want to do everything yourself, cannot delegate
  – Not being able to say no
  – Always want to be there for others

- Allowing the unexpected to be imposed on you again and again
- Excessive search for recognition
- False ambition
- Fear of "emptiness", of "doing nothing", of boredom
- Want to be accessible to everyone at any time, in any place
- Other: ...
- **Scheduling errors**
  - Delayed start
  - Dwelling on unimportant things, no clear priorities
  - Excessive working hours
  - Failure to complete a job
  - Missing or too late closing point
  - Waiver of breaks
  - Hasty and therefore faulty work
  - Frequent switching from one work in progress to another
  - Too tight a schedule, no room for the unexpected
  - Underestimating the time needed for individual tasks
  - "Mania for order" or defective order
  - Other: ...

Everyday stressors often also arise in the interpersonal sphere, that is from interaction with other people in the family, at work, and in leisure time. Such **relationship stressors** consist, for example, in psychosocial conflicts and tensions that one does not know how to resolve, a lack of recognition, experienced rejection or injustice. A lack of social contact, that is loneliness can become a severe stressor, as can social overstimulation when there is too much social contact, as is the case in some service occupations. Here are some examples of such interpersonal stressors: you are confronted with complaints from customers or accusations from your supervisor and do not know how to respond. You experience strong competitive behaviour from colleagues and cannot stand up to it. You have disappointments, breakups or losses to deal with, or live in a chronic conflict situation that you cannot resolve. You are overwhelmed with high, possibly difficult to reconcile, expectations from other members of your family that you cannot meet.

Relationship stressors

It is of great importance that stress reactions can be triggered not only by the real confrontation with the stressors but also by their mental anticipation. Unpleasant events cast their shadows in advance. Stress is triggered by the mental preoc-

Mental preoccupation with difficult situations as stress triggers

3

cupation with future difficult situations. Exam anxiety is a classic example of this. Not only the real loss of one's job but also the fear of losing one's job represents a burden that triggers physical and mental stress reactions.

It is especially these—real or anticipated—performance-related and interpersonal demands that determine the stress experience of many people today. They are not so much a threat to vital physical needs, but rather to central psychological motives for love and recognition, for security, for contact and belonging, for self-realization and self-esteem. And, like physical stressors, they trigger intense physical and psychological stress responses that activate us and mobilize our energy to escape the threat, avert harm, and compensate for loss. We often succeed in this in one way or another. We find ways to restore our balance. The stress reactions come to an end and we have learned something new. New behaviours that we can fall back on in the future when we face similar threatening situations. Ultimately, the stress episode has helped us develop and improve our skills.

When coping fails...   But what about when the defense against the threat fails, when we—no matter how hard we try—cannot find a solution? Then the arousal remains. We enter a state of continuous stress. This is especially likely when we are confronted with major life-changing events and strokes of fate that, in a sense, shake up our entire lives over a long period of time, or when everyday stressors in our work and personal lives persist or recur over a long period of time without giving us enough time to recover. It is these chronic performance-related and interpersonal stressors, in particular, that define the stress experience of many people today. And it is, in particular, the chronic stress reactions, that is, those that are maintained over a long period of time and can no longer be down-regulated, that endanger the physical and mental health of many people today (▶ Sect. 2.9).

3.3 Societal Roots: Looking Beyond the Horizon

Western societies have been experiencing a fundamental change in the world of work for well over two decades. Globalization, flexibilization, digitalization, virtualization, and privatization are buzzwords for these far-reaching changes that are affecting our working world and, beyond that, all other areas of our lives.

Dealing with the stressors inevitably also leads us to reflect on these societal changes, which play a decisive role in shaping the spectrum of stressors we are confronted with today. Such reflection on the societal dimension of the stress phenomenon can help us to better understand our personal stressful life situations and lead to the relieving realization that many people share our experiences of stress and are faced with similar demands to master as oneself. We recognize ourselves and our lives as part of a larger whole, embedded in social structures and developments. In the remainder of this chapter, I would, therefore, like to shed light on at least some of the social developments that shape many people's experience of stress today.

I have repeatedly emphasized that stress is essentially a highly individual process in which personal goals, motives, attitudes, and behaviour play a significant role. However, it would be too short-sighted if we were to view stress exclusively and unilaterally as the personal problem of each individual. After all, the demands we face every day are largely not determined by the individual himself, but have their origin in the social conditions in which we live our lives. Social conditions shape the professional, educational, and also private worlds of life, each with its own specific pattern of demands that have to be mastered. And what is more: social conditions not only shape the external demands, but also our personal motives, attitudes, and behaviours with which we approach these demands and which can act as personal stress amplifiers. Through upbringing, we internalize the norms, values, and standards of behaviour of the society in which we live. We are children of our time. So if we want to talk about stress and understand stress, we also need to think about the social conditions that shape stress-producing demands and personal stress-amplifying behaviours.

Looking beyond the horizon of our own stressful everyday life to the societal background can help us to better understand and classify our personal stress experiences. And it can contribute to a relieving, relativizing, and accepting view of our personal everyday stress. It is not about complaining about how bad the world is or has become, but about perceiving changes and recognizing that new competencies are required in order to be able to lead one's own life in balance in the changing world. At the same time, reflecting on the social background also opens our eyes to the necessity of working within our own sphere of influence and responsibility for such working and living conditions in which a life in a healthy balance of tension and relaxation becomes possible in the first place.

Societal dimension of stress

Classify personal stress experiences

3

3.4 Stress at Work: The New Work Creates New Demands

Change of work

Work intensification, acceleration, and increased competition in globalized markets characterize everyday life in many companies. The compulsion to increase productivity has resulted in an ever greater compression and intensification of work. Work is becoming more intensive, more complex and takes up more time. Operating on global markets and the introduction of modern means of communication lead to a delimitation of working hours and working locations. Work is possible and often demanded at any time and in any place. Discontinuous employment biographies with more frequent job changes, temporary employment contracts, and periods without employment characterize the working lives of more and more people and often create an existential feeling of insecurity.

From industrial work to service

Hand in hand with the continuing globalized division of labour, we are also experiencing a change in work itself, a change away from industrial work towards information work and services. The speed at which these changes are taking place is enormous and unprecedented in human history. For 3.5 million years, man was a hunter-gatherer, for more than 10,000 years a farmer and craftsman, for almost 200 years an industrial worker—and for about two decades now he has been predominantly a service provider and "information worker". Classic industrial jobs in the manufacturing sector now account for only about 30% of all jobs. According to statistics from the Federal Association of Company Health Insurance Funds in Germany, the proportion of members employed in manufacturing and construction has fallen by about half, from just under 75% in 1978 to about 34% in 2005. At the same time, the number of members in service sectors such as commerce, credit, insurance, administration, health, and social services has risen from 22% in 1978 to over 50% in 2005.

Stressors at the workplace

With the transition from an industrial to a service society, the stressors at the workplace have also changed. It is no longer the beat of the machine, heavy physical work, dust, noise, heat, cold, or draughts that are the primary health hazards. Instead, more and more employees find an excessive workload, increasing time pressure and the fear of losing their job stressful. Modern communication technologies and operating in globalized markets require a high degree of local mobility and time flexibility on the part of employees.

Living with uncertainty

At the same time, forms of corporate management and work organization are also changing. Direct forms of control ("command and control") are increasingly being replaced by indirect, results-oriented forms of control ("management by objectives"). In this case, the performance of employees is assessed solely on the basis of the results achieved; the duration and manner of performance as well as any problems that may have arisen in the process are irrelevant to the assessment and are the sole responsibility of the employee. Flexible working hours, performance-related pay, and management by objectives are prominent features of such a form of indirect results-oriented corporate management. This requires increased personal responsibility and self-organization on the part of the employees.

The rapid pace of technological progress demands a willingness to engage in lifelong learning. The knowledge and skills acquired during vocational training or studies are no longer sufficient for an entire working life. The compulsion to increase productivity in globalized competition means that every single employee has to be more willing to perform and more competitive. At the same time, work is becoming more insecure. The fear of losing one's job and of social decline is increasing. The days of starting as an apprentice in a company and then continuing to work in the same profession until retirement is definitely over. We have to learn to live with this new uncertainty and need to find security and stability within ourselves. How this can be achieved will be one of the topics of the second part of this book.

3.5 Resource or Burden: The Two Faces of Work

» It is a double face that carries the work. It contains both a curse and a blessing. It is up to us to take the sting out of work, to shape it in such a way that we can enjoy its blessings without increasing the suffering and hardship of life. (Emil Kraepelin, German psychiatrist, 1856–1926)

Due to the great importance of work not only for securing one's livelihood but also for the formation of one's identity in modern societies, stress experiences associated with gainful employment play a prominent role in psychological well-being and physical health. The great importance of work for one's own physical and psychological well-being is often only fully realized when one no longer has a job. Work is not just about earning a living and thus securing one's material existence, but also makes an essential contribution to satisfying fundamental human needs and motives. Work helps us to structure our everyday life. Through work we come into contact with other people and experience a sense of belonging. We experience

Work conveys meaning and inner stability

3

Stress factors at the workplace

recognition and self-affirmation. We test and develop our abilities and skills. Work gives us a sense of identity and purpose. In this sense, work is a very central resource for the psychological stability and health of the individual. This is especially true in societies like ours, where work/occupation/achievement is generally accepted to be of great importance.

On the other hand, there are the work stressors that can lead to a risk to physical and mental health. These can result from the work tasks themselves, the material and social working conditions and the organization of work. Since the mid-1980s, an increase in mental stress has been observed in the world of work, while physical stressors have decreased in importance.

Psychological stress on the rise

Employee surveys in a wide variety of industries repeatedly show that many employees experience the way in which work tasks are organized, structured, and communicated as stressful, rather than the work tasks as such. A maximum of 30–40% of the stress factors relate to the work tasks as such and the physical-material working conditions. 60–70% of the stress factors, on the other hand, have to do with the organization of work as well as with psycho-mental and social aspects of work. And: stress caused by physical-material factors at the workplace (noise, cold or heat …) is usually experienced as less severe than stress caused by problems in the organizational and social area. To put it bluntly: a bad office chair or a bad room climate is more easily endured by most employees than a superior who is experienced as unfair or a bad working atmosphere.

Psychosocial stressors in the workplace

Common psychosocial stressors cited in the workplace include:

- high time pressure or too much work in the time available,
- lack of or insufficient information from superiors and colleagues,
- unclear or constantly increasing targets,
- lack of recognition of performance (no positive feedback),
- injustices experienced, promises not kept,
- being overwhelmed with tasks without being able to set your own priorities,
- no or too few conversations,
- unforeseen changes in the work situation without prior consultation and preparation,
- lack of understanding from superiors and colleagues for difficulties in the professional and also private sphere.

> ❯ **Important**
> To sum up: the prevailing stressors in the world of work today consist in
> 1. excessive demands on performance due to an increasing workload, which manifests itself in work and time pressure and
> 2. in the organizational and social working conditions, through which central needs for security, for belonging, for recognition and self-affirmation are not or not sufficiently fulfilled or are threatened.

To Think Further
- What changes (e.g. introduction of new technologies, restructuring, relocation of production sites, redundancies, changes in organization and management, etc.) have you experienced in your workplace in recent years?
- What impact have these changes had on your work and daily life?
- What do you think of these changes?

In recent years, occupational scientists have presented extensive studies in which they examined the characteristics of particularly stressful workplaces in even greater detail.

Workplaces at particular risk of stress

▪ High Demands and Little Scope for Decision-Making

According to the "demand-control model" of the two Swedish stress researchers Richard Karasek and Töres Theorell, workplaces particularly at risk of stress are characterized by a combination of high quantitative work demands (especially as a result of time pressure) on the one hand and a low degree of control over the work process or little scope for decision-making at the workplace on the other. The person concerned is unable to process his tasks in an active and success-controlled manner and experiences that he is unable to control essential aspects of his environment. A classic example of this is assembly line work, but such a constellation also exists in many low-status office and service occupations. As relevant scientific studies have shown, holders of such jobs are 2–4 times more at risk of developing cardiovascular disease prematurely, that is between the ages of 35 and 65, regardless of their hereditary or behavioural risk. The risk of developing a depressive disorder is doubled.

Little control

If there is additionally a lack of social support at the workplace from colleagues and superiors, that is if employees have the feeling that they are left alone when problems arise and

Lack of support

3

perceive a lack of positive team spirit, the risk of illness increases further. The more the work pressure increases, the more important it is to give employees room for manoeuvre and decision-making and to offer reliable social support in order to prevent stress-related illnesses and burnout. Both factors act as a buffer, so to speak, which can protect against the harmful effects on health of increasing work and time pressure.

- **Lack of Reward for High Commitment**

Low reward

In his **"Effort-reward-imbalance-model"** the German medical sociologist Johannes Siegrist does not focus on the aspect of the controllability of a work task, but on the reward granted for a work performance rendered. Siegrist describes a discrepancy between high effort spent at work on the one hand and low reward received on the other as a stress-producing gratification crisis, which can lead to serious health disorders. Rewards for performance do not consist solely in wages or salary, but also in particular in the recognition and appreciation that the employee experiences at his or her workplace, as well as in career advancement opportunities and job security.

High effort

On the one hand, high levels of effort can be caused by external demands (e.g. as a result of time pressure), on the other hand, they can also be based on an individual's excessive work-related commitment ("overcommitment"). This refers to the tendency of certain people to identify without distance with the demands placed on them, which leads to performance expectations and rewards being assessed unrealistically: Affected individuals often perform better than is expected of them. A prospective study of industrial workers found a three- to four-fold increased risk of heart attack in individuals who exhibited both high levels of effort and low opportunities for gratification. If there were also known physical risk factors (obesity, elevated blood pressure, elevated LDL cholesterol), the probability of suffering a heart attack during the 6-year observation period increased to up to 85%. Further international studies show that the combination of high expenditure and low reward increases the risk of cardiovascular disease by 2–4 times and of depressive disorders by 2–3 times.

Reward through appreciation

The more the demands of work increase, the more important it becomes to ensure appropriate rewards for the work performed in order to prevent stress-related illnesses and burnout. This is not just about money, but also about social recognition, appreciation, and security. In contrast to praise and recognition, appreciation is independent of the actual work performance and instead relates to the employee as an individual person. Companies have many ways of expressing such personal appreciation to their employees. These range from a pleasant design of work spaces and resources to offers that make it easier for individuals to reconcile work and family, to an appreciative approach by managers to their employees, which also includes an interest in the personal concerns of employees. This last point in particular, the leadership culture in a company and the specific leadership behaviour of managers have a major influence on the stress experience of employees, both negatively and positively. Another important source of gratification is the guarantee of a stable livelihood in the long term. In the modern world of work, this is no longer the case, or not to a sufficient degree, for more and more people. Job insecurity and fear of losing one's job are a burden on many people. This is probably one of the main causes of the gratification crises described by Siegrist, with their serious health effects.

■ **Burnout in Companies**

The two American organizational psychologists Christina Maslach and Michael Leiter have conducted extensive research into the causes of the burnout syndrome (▶ Sect. 2.10). In their book "The Truth about Burnout" they identify six structural conditions of the modern working world that can lead to long-lasting stress and ultimately to burnout not only of individual employees but also of entire work teams and company units. These conditions are:

Structural conditions for burnout

— Work overload,
— Lack of control,
— Insufficient reward,
— The collapse of the community,
— Lack of fairness, and
— Contradictory values.

The first four of Maslach and Leiter's burnout factors are already familiar to us from work stress models. The last two factors, lack of fairness and conflicting values, undermine the individual employee's commitment to his or her work as well as his or her identification with the company and, according to Maslach and Leiter, lead directly to burnout. Unfair situations, such as when individuals are favoured by participating in special events, pay differentials, or different treatment of vacation requests, are experienced as very stressful by others who witness it. Terminations are also extremely stressful for the rest of the team, especially when they occur for reasons that cannot be understood. Everyone fears for their job. Who will be the next one? For example, a study by Finnish occupational physician Jussi Vahtera among municipal employees showed that workers who experience colleagues being laid off have a significantly increased risk of dying from heart disease in the following 4 years.

Lack of fairness

3

> In summary, it can be stated that particularly stressful jobs can be characterized by a combination of high quantitative and/or qualitative demands with, only low decision latitude, a lack of social support at the workplace, and a lack of recognition of work performance and personal appreciation.

Stress prevention in the workplace

The results of work stress research provide important indications for stress prevention and stress management measures in the workplace. They make it clear that for effective prevention of stress-related health risks in the world of work, it is not enough simply to promote the coping skills of individual employees to deal with new demands by means of appropriate training programmes. In addition, structural measures are also required which are aimed at a health-promoting design of work tasks and processes as well as of organizational and social-communicative conditions (management style) at the workplace. Individual and structural stress management must go hand in hand here.

3.6 Stress in the Family: The Support Givers Become Weaker

Family as a support

For most people, partnership and family are sources of strength and support. There they experience security. They feel accepted just as they are. They can let themselves go and recharge their batteries. Shared experiences of physical and emotional closeness and trust form a real protective mantle against which the stresses of everyday life are buffered. Physical contact, tenderness, and sexuality lower the level of stress hormones and create a deep feeling of relaxation and well-being. On the other hand, however, strong stress can also arise in emotionally significant relationships, when conflicts smoulder and quarrels determine everyday life. Scientific studies show that the loss of a partner or the separation from a partner are the events with the highest stress value of all.

Disintegration of social ties

Private relationships are also affected by the profound changes in the world of work. Hand in hand with the economic changes, an increasing dissolution of tradition-determined family social ties can be observed. Sociologists say that we live in a society that strives less for ties than for options, a society in which so-called weak ties have gained in importance, especially in the world of work, and so-called strong ties to family and kinship have lost considerable stability and continuity. The high number of one-person households, still decreasing numbers of children as well as increasing divorce rates are unmistakable signs of this social development.

The mobility requirements of the modern working world make it difficult to maintain relationships with partners and a constant family life. Spending time together is often only possible through complicated appointment arrangements. For daily and weekly commuters, their role in the family is changing. It is not unusual for them to feel like a guest in their own home at the weekend. They are largely excluded from the everyday life of the family.

The (over)emphasis on work and performance in our society is linked to a disregard for the care and upbringing of children. Children represent one of the most important poverty risks in our society, as social and income statistics and the German Federal Government's poverty report state year after year. The low social standing and poor material conditions put a strain on the already demanding task of bringing up children. Last but not least, insufficient and qualitatively inadequate childcare facilities make it difficult to reconcile family and work and cause a variety of daily burdens in families, which are not only of an organizational nature but also of an emotional nature (feelings of guilt). The so-called reconciliation management (which, by the way, is still all too often left to women alone), the daily struggle to reconcile one's own professional and career goals with the different needs of the family members, not only requires a high degree of organization, planning, and often improvization, but also places high demands on the communication, compromise, and conflict skills of the life partners.

Reconciliation of work and family life

Caring for sick and elderly family members also places enormous financial, organizational and, above all, emotional burdens on caring relatives, which often take them to their own limits and can become an ordeal for the whole family.

Caring for relatives

The erosion of traditional social relationships is not limited to the close family circle, but also extends to other established social structures such as kinship, neighbourhood and circles of friends. The mobility requirements of the modern working world demand a repeated willingness to move one's centre of life to where the work is. This promotes social insecurity, role confusion, and loneliness and places high demands on the social skills of the individual, who must repeatedly establish a new social network. This further increases the pressure on the nuclear family. In the absence of other social relationships, all contact and communication needs are projected onto the life partner. Mutual disappointments are virtually pre-programmed. Where the nuclear family is not integrated into another social network, it alone must withstand the pressure of everyday small and large burdens. Many a partnership is overwhelmed by this and breaks up, also because the partners neglect to nurture their relationship in time, carefully and regularly in order to give it the necessary stability.

Strains on the partner relationship

In terms of social policy, it is of the utmost importance to strengthen the family as an important support for the individual in an increasingly uncertain world. In particular, it is a matter of enabling the compatibility of family and career through appropriate financial and legal framework conditions, through sufficient childcare and care services, through family-friendly working conditions and hours and, last but not least, through a change in thinking in our child-deprived, overly one-sided performance-fixated society.

3.7   Stress in Leisure Time: How Recovery Fails

Disturbed work-life balance

Leisure time is also influenced by the change in work. First work, then pleasure—in this credo of the Protestant work ethic, work is given clear priority, but at least pleasure still occurs and there is a life alongside work. In the modern world of work, this sounds strangely old-fashioned, antiquated, and outdated. For more and more people, including dependent employees, not just freelancers and the self-employed, "work is actually never over". The conventional structuring of the daily routine into working time on the one hand and free time on the other is increasingly dissolving in the modern service society. Constant availability for the customer is demanded and made possible by technological developments such as the mobile phone and the Internet. Working is possible anytime and anywhere. If rigidly prescribed working hours are relaxed, this means that the individual can—and must—decide to a greater extent about his or her own time, or at least about how to allocate it. This is associated with no small demand on planning and organizational skills, the so-called self-management skills. Many people feel overwhelmed by these demands for self-organization and fail to draw a clear line between work and leisure in their everyday lives, with the long-term fatal result that "free time" no longer exists as the counterweight to work that is so important for regeneration. The balance between work and leisure, the so-called work-life balance, is disturbed.

"Recreational stress"

There is a remarkable contradiction here: statistically speaking, we have more and more free time. This is not only due to the reduction in working hours in recent decades, but also due to technical achievements that make time-consuming household chores easier or take them away completely. At the same time, more and more people are complaining about time constraints and hectic schedules, even in their free time. A representative survey conducted by the Cologne Sports University under the direction of psychologist Henning Allmer revealed that 75% of Germans are unable to relax in their free time. How does this contradiction come about? There is a widespread disdain in our society for "free" time as a free space for non-purposeful activity. Norms and criteria of the working world are transferred to leisure time. Performance thinking, perfectionism, ambition, prestige, and the need to consume all too often determine leisure behaviour. Hectic activity, impatience, and the fear of missing out leave no room for inner peace and leisure, for "doing nothing". Thus, often leisure time is not a regenerative counter-world to working life, but rather its duplication.

3.8 Stress due to Uncertainty: The Pleasure and Burden of Choice

Not only social life contexts, but also socially or ecclesiastically and religiously shaped structures of meaning and values are losing their binding force. Traditions give less and less support and orientation to fewer and fewer people. In our open society, there is a pluralism of values and a wide range of religious or ideological offers of meaning.

Traditions dissolve

This opens up the opportunity for each individual to have a greater degree of self-determination in the shaping and planning of his or her own life. Whereas in earlier times, the individual's way of life was dictated by traditions and norms, today we are allowed and obliged to make our own decisions. This begins with everyday things such as the choice of clothing, haircut, and diet continues with existential decisions such as the choice of profession, the choice of life partner and the way in which we live together, the decision on the number of children and the time and method of their birth, and ends with the choice of one's own religion or world view and the determination of the rite according to which one's own funeral should take place. The open society offers at any time a variety of options, between which we may choose and—and here the philosopher Wilhelm Schmid sees a dilemma of modern freedom of choice—also must choose. Freedom of choice becomes a necessity.

Chance of self-determination

This places high demands on individual decision-making and judgment. Those who have to find their own way need an inner compass, their own goals, and inner independence. We may and must choose, but can we? Quite a few people feel overwhelmed by the great freedom of choice. They experience the freedom of choice above all as uncertainty. They find it difficult to make decisions according to their own goals and priorities. Some try to keep all their options open, driving

The "agony of choice"

3

themselves into overload. The more options a person has, the more she wants to realize, the less she wants to lose, the more she charges herself, the less time remains in the end. She tries to pack two lives into one for fear of missing the decisive one.

Work as a source of meaning

For many other people, the loss of traditional ties and the accompanying uncertainty mean that work, performance, and professional success remain as the sole criteria that determine their place and value in society, and often represent the last and only reliable crystallization point for inner stability, for the formation of one's own identity, and sense of purpose. For more and more people, the following is increasingly true: I am what I achieve—in the eyes of other people as well as in front of myself.

Thus, on the one hand, work is subjectively becoming more and more important for the individual as a source of meaning and support; on the other hand, work is simultaneously becoming more insecure. In order to reduce insecurity, many people react to this by concentrating their lives even more on work. But this has fatal consequences. In the absence of work, for example, through retirement, job cuts or illness and other, sources of support such as family, friendships, faith, etc. are missing. This triggers deep crises of meaning, depression, and health disorders.

3.9   Severe Life Stress: Does Misfortune Make You Ill?

Major life events as stressors

In addition to the chronic stressors of work and everyday life, drastic life events represent a class of stressors in their own right. Attentive physicians have always made the observation that the onset of a physical illness or mental disorder is often temporally related to the occurrence of serious life-changing events, such as a divorce or separation, a job change or loss, children moving out, etc. A particularly glaring example is retirement death, which some people, especially those who are professionally engaged, die within a short time of retirement. The most stressful life event for most people is the death of their life partner. Not infrequently as a consequence, the widowed partner who is left behind falls ill and even dies within the year of mourning.

The effect of major life events and strokes of fate on health has been investigated in a large number of scientific studies. The basic idea is that readjustment after such critical life events entails intense stress for the person concerned, which triggers strong stress reactions that can in turn trigger and/or intensify illness. As early as 1967, the two American scientists

☐ Table 3.1 Selection of life-changing events with stress point values. (Adapted from Holmes and Rahe 1967)

Life event	Stress points
Death of the spouse	100
Divorce	73
Legal separation	65
Death of a close relative	63
Severe physical injury or illness	53
Marriage	50
Termination by the employer	47
Retirement	45
Pregnancy	40
Change to other work	36
Children move out	29
Change of residence	25
Difficulties with superiors	23
Change of residence	20
Change of school	20

Holmes and Rahe developed a scale with a total of 43 different critical life events. Based on their research findings, they assigned a specific stress point value to each of these events. The death of a life partner has the highest stress point value of 100 and is classified, for example, as four times as serious as a change of residence (☐ Table 3.1). The point value increases with the number of life events, and with it the risk of illness. It is particularly serious if several drastic life events have to be coped with simultaneously or in quick succession, which is unfortunately often the case.

However, the results of life event research also make it clear that—just as with everyday stressors—it is not so much the occurrence of the event itself as its perception, evaluation, and processing by the person affected that is decisive in determining whether or not health disorders subsequently occur. Events such as a change of school, a move and even the death of a close relative can have very different individual meanings. They can be experienced as a threat or loss, but also as a challenge or even redemption. How strong the physical stress reactions are and whether or not health disorders occur as a result depends on a large extent on the subjective significance of the

Valuation decisive

3

event. The subjective processes of processing potentially stressful events will be discussed in detail in the following chapter.

3.10 Checklist: Personal Stress Hierarchy

Personal stressor hierarchy

In ◘ Fig. 3.1, you will find a list of common stressors in work and everyday life. Please check which of these stressors occur in your personal everyday life. Then go through these individual stressors again and consider how heavy each stressor weighs in your everyday life. Weight the burdens that you have marked with "Yes" with a point value: You have a total of 10 points available, which you can distribute among the various burdens according to their severity. Of course, you can also—in extreme cases—assign all 10 points to one burden. The other burdens then receive no points. In this way, you obtain a ranking of your most important stress factors.

Everyday stressors			
In my everyday life I feel burdened by			
	Yes	No	Points
Deadline pressure, time constraints, rushing			
Difficulties in combining work and private life			
Family obligations (e.g. in the household, care of relatives, child care)			
Dissatisfaction with the distribution of housework			
Social/voluntary commitments (e.g., in clubs or organizations)			
Health problems (e.g., illnesses, consequences of illnesses, or chronic conditions) in myself or others			
Long commutes to work or frequent business trips			
Marital or partnership conflicts			
Problems with children (e.g., parenting or school)			
Financial worries (e.g. unemployment, installment payments)			
High responsibility at work (e.g., great risk of causing harm)			
Dissatisfaction with my job (e.g., being underchallenged, bored, too routine)			
Dissatisfaction with my working conditions or hours (e.g., noise, heat, constantly changing work hours)			
Disruptions in daily work (e.g., constant interruptions or poor planning)			
Constant accessibility (through email, cell phone, etc.)			
Different demands at work that I cannot meet at the same time			
High workload/work pace			

☐ **Fig. 3.1** Checklist: Everyday stressors

3

	Yes	No	Points
Introduction of new working methods and technologies			
Information overload or lack of information			
Personal tensions at work (e.g. with colleagues, superiors or customers)			
Lack of appreciation and recognition of one's own work performance			
Disagreements within the circle of relatives			
Frequently recurring disputes with other people (e.g. landlords, tenants or neighbors)			
Dissatisfaction with living situation (e.g. noise, apartment too small, poor location, etc.)			
Timing of daily routine (e.g., too little or too much free time, too little sleep)			
Fear of an imminent deterioration of the existing life situation (e.g. due to unemployment or illness)			
Other (here you can name further burdens)			

Evaluation:
Go through the individual burdens again and consider how heavy each burden weighs in your everyday life. Weight the burdens that you have checked with "Yes" with a point value:
You have a total of 10 points available, which you can distribute among the various burdens according to their severity. Of course, you can also - in extreme cases - assign all 10 points to one load. The other burdens will then not receive any points. In this way, you obtain a ranking of your burdens.

My personal hierarchy of daily stressors

1. _____

2. _____

3. _____

4. _____

5. _____

☐ **Fig. 3.1** (continued)

Personal Stress Amplifiers: How We Put Ourselves Under Stress

Contents

© Springer-Verlag GmbH Germany, part of Springer Nature 2022
G. Kaluza, *Calm and Confident Under Stress*, https://doi.org/10.1007/978-3-662-64440-9_4

4

» It is not the things or events themselves that worry us, but the attitudes and opinions we have about things. (Epictetus, Greek philosopher of the Stoa, 50-138 A.D.)

To a considerable extent, stress arises in the mind: by the way, we perceive and evaluate demands and our own competencies. By the extent to which we attribute personal significance for our self-esteem and for our inner balance to the requirements and see ourselves personally threatened by a possible failure. By the glasses through which we perceive things, for example, whether we perceive mainly negative/threatening aspects, risks, and our own deficits or also see positive aspects, opportunities, and our own strengths. To the extent to which we get caught up in unnecessary ruminations about past situations ("Why did this happen to me? If only I had paid more attention ...") or exaggerated worries about future situations ("What will come of it? What if I fail? ..."). All of this plays a decisive role in whether or not we will experience stress at all in a given situation and how intense und long-lasting our stress experience will be.

This also means: we are not passively exposed to the stressors in our environment, but we actively relate ourselves to given demands. Here, mental processes in the form of evaluative perceptions, expectations, and conclusions play the decisive role. In this chapter, we will deal in detail with these subjective processes of individual stress processing.

4.1 Stress is the Result of Personal Evaluations

Basically, we can distinguish between two different appraisal processes that are decisive for whether or not the biological stress system is triggered:

1. Appraisal of the situation
   Evaluations that include an assessment of the situation or the respective requirements. Requirements can be assessed either as neutral-irrelevant, as pleasant-positive or as threatening-harmful. A stress-related evaluation occurs when requirements are assessed as threatening or harmful, that is when the person sees important personal motives and goals endangered, attacked, or violated by the requirement. These include the achievement motive ("I want to perform well"), the affiliation motive ("I want to belong"), and the autonomy motive ("I want to decide for myself"). The more pronounced such motives are, the more important it becomes for one's own balance and self-esteem that these motives are actually fulfilled. And the more sensitively a wide variety of situations will be appraised as pos-

sible threats to these personal motives and responded to accordingly with stress reactions. Therefore, the crucial question here is: what actually does make a requirement or its successful coping personally important to me, with which "personal shares" am I invested in this situation?

2. Appraisal of coping options
   Assessments that include an evaluation of one's own coping skills and possibilities. Here, one's own competencies in dealing with the respective requirement are assessed as well as external support options that can be used to cope with the requirement, if necessary. These can be assessed as either sufficient or insufficient for successful coping with the requirements. In the second case, there is a stress-related evaluation. Obviously, past experiences with coping with demand situations play an important role in this evaluation process. These may have shaped general attitudes of one's own helplessness which now also take effect in the current situation. Alternatively, previous experience may have strengthened optimistic confidence in one's own abilities, which leads to confidence in one's ability to cope with the current, new challenge.

An Example

Let us try to illustrate these evaluation processes with an example (◻ Fig. 4.1). Please try to imagine the following situation as vividly as possible: it is a completely normal working day in a completely normal working week. Completely unexpectedly you are called to your boss. He assigns you a new task that has to be completed within the next week. On your way out, your boss mentions how important this task is for the department and that he is counting on you.

This is a situation that probably occurs in many offices or workshops. Whether or not and how strongly stress reactions are triggered in this situation will largely depend on how you mentally adjust to the situation. You may have experienced such situations frequently in the past and handled them well. You see such special assignments as part of your job. Your evaluation of the situation tends to be neutral to irrelevant, because you are sure that you will be able to cope with the new task as you have done in the past. Perhaps, however, you have been waiting for a chance to show what you are made of and to escape the normal work routine that has made you dissatisfied for a long time. You are glad that your boss has chosen you. The situation is more of a pleasant-positive challenge for you. You trust in your abilities and that you will learn what you cannot yet do.

Example: Individual appraisal processes

4

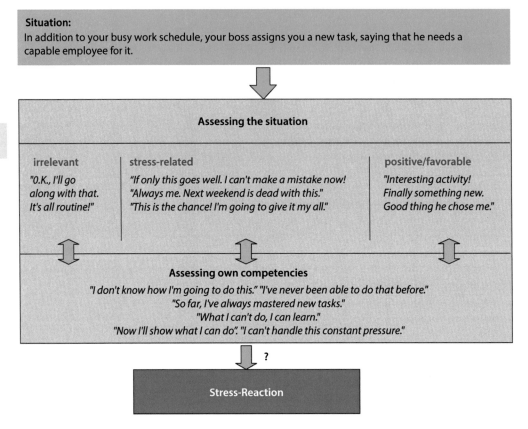

Situation:
In addition to your busy work schedule, your boss assigns you a new task, saying that he needs a capable employee for it.

Assessing the situation

irrelevant	stress-related	positive/favorable
"O.K., I'll go along with that. It's all routine!"	"If only this goes well. I can't make a mistake now! "Always me. Next weekend is dead with this." "This is the chance! I'm going to give it my all."	"Interesting activity! Finally something new. Good thing he chose me."

Assessing own competencies
"I don't know how I'm going to do this." "I've never been able to do that before."
"So far, I've always mastered new tasks."
"What I can't do, I can learn."
"Now I'll show what I can do". "I can't handle this constant pressure."

?

Stress-Reaction

◻ Fig. 4.1   Stress is the result of personal evaluations (example)

Challenge vs. threat

It is also possible, however, that your thoughts revolve primarily around how you can win the recognition of the boss, which is so important to you, and how terrible it would be for you if you disappoint him. Or you are struggling with the fact that the extra work will overshadow the planned weekend with the family. The situation has more of a threatening to damaging character for you. You torture yourself with thoughts of how you are going to manage it all and withstand the pressure.

Obviously, we are dealing here with quite different mental assessments of one and the same situation. Which of these assessments is "correct" or "true"? There is no answer to this question. There is no objectively correct or only one true view of things here. Rather, each of the views described has a subjective truth for the person concerned, insofar as they reflect personal previous experiences with similar situations as well as one's own goals and motives, that is in our example career goals, the desire for recognition or for a quiet weekend.

Of course, the assessments of the situation and one's own coping options can be more or less in line with reality. It is possible that we are actually faced with high demands for which we lack the necessary competencies, skills, or knowledge to be able to cope successfully. Then we are, in a sense, rightly under stress. In this case, it is not a matter of "thinking positively" about the situation or of telling ourselves that we do have the necessary skills. This would not be helpful in terms of successfully coping with the demands of the situation, and would probably also not be very helpful in terms of regulating one's own tension. Often, however, there is no objective yardstick. Many of the performance-related and social situations we are confronted with every day are ambiguous and leave room for personal interpretation and evaluation. These can be distorted in a stress-exacerbating manner, resulting in activation of the biological stress program in a variety of situations. We then speak of stress aggravating thought patterns and personal stress amplifiers. These will be discussed in the following.

> **Conclusion**
> To summarize up to this point: A stress-related evaluation of requirements is present if we
> 1. Assess the requirement as subjectively significant, that is we see important areas of life, needs, motives, and goals threatened or damaged by the situation in question and
> 2. Consider our own competencies and the available external resources to be insufficient for successfully meeting the requirement

4.2 Stress Aggravating Thought Patterns

How should one approach the demands of work and everyday life mentally in order to get into stress as often and as intensively as possible? Let us take a look at this question and try, even if it sounds paradoxical in the context of this book, to formulate some recommendations for stress-intensifying thinking.

» **"This can't be true!" thinking**

When we are faced with demands, difficult, or unpleasant situations, we refuse to accept them as reality. Instead, we resent the fact that the situation is the way it is. For example, we are stuck in a traffic jam or in a long line at the department store checkout, so our schedule gets thrown off. We face an unexpected difficulty in completing a work task because we our-

Struggling with reality

4

selves or one of our colleagues or co-workers missed something. We missed an important ball while playing golf, soccer, tennis, or volleyball. We hit a bump while parking. A client pulls out of a big order at the last moment. In these and similar situations, we give as much room as possible in our brains to one thought: "This can't be true!" This thought will reliably increase anger and physical activation in us. We can really get caught up in stress and anger with this thought, and it will prevent us from dealing constructively with the situation at hand to make the best of it. This thought is also particularly effective when we apply it to our own unpleasant or unwanted reactions. For example, when we stutter or blush in a conversation, when we get a dry mouth in a presentation, or when our hands shake. Because what cannot be cannot be, the "No way!" thought leads us further into anger or anxiety and tension. We then experience anger over anger, fear over fear, and excitement over excitement.

Denying reality

Yet another variant of this stress-exacerbating thought pattern is to be addressed here: the not wanting to be true in the sense of a downright denial of reality. The focus here is not on struggling with what is, but on ignoring, fading out, simply not taking note of a situation. This is a psychological defense mechanism that protects us from being overwhelmed by overly painful feelings of fear or grief in the face of serious threats or losses, such as being told of a serious illness diagnosis or the death of a loved one. In the short term, denial brings relief, but when maintained over time, it prevents us from actively dealing with the situation.

» View of the negative

Negative generalization

This is a quite simple and at the same time extremely effective strategy to put ourselves under stress. We do this by selectively focusing our attention on the negative events of a day or the negative aspects of a situation. We give these negative experiences an outsized importance, losing any reasonable standard and blanking out positive experiences. A critical comment from a supervisor, spouse or colleague, a failed cake, a blown appointment, a dent in the car, an unfortunate conversation with an acquaintance can then, if we only give these events the right amount of importance, ruin our entire day. We then generalize these negative experiences as broadly as possible with thoughts such as "I just can't do it", "I'm a bad housewife", "Nothing ever works out", "The car is total crap", "Nobody likes me". With such thoughts in our minds, we then mentally set ourselves up to reliably experience stress, anger, and frustration throughout the rest of the day.

■ **Negative Consequences Thinking**

When we think about an upcoming challenge, such as an exam, an important negotiation with a client, or a medical operation, we focus our attention as exclusively as possible on the negative consequences of failing to meet the challenge. We picture the failure and the catastrophic negative consequences, it will have in great detail, recall previous negative experiences if necessary, and avoid as much as possible any thought of a successful outcome and the positive consequences associated with it. We also consistently keep thoughts of how we have successfully mastered similar situations in the past and what skills we have demonstrated or acquired in the process away from our consciousness. *In* this way, we will reliably cause intense feelings of stress and physical stress reactions in advance. In the situation itself, it is then very likely that exactly what we have constantly feared beforehand will occur, namely failure. In competitive sports, this strategy is well known. Some athletes are world champions in training. They can actually do it. It is just that when it comes down to it, in competition, they cannot perform to their full potential. They think about the possible negative consequences of defeat, which makes them nervous and tense and reduces their performance.

Painting negative consequences

■ **Personalize**

By this is meant, above all, that we take events and behaviours of others as personally as possible. We feel that we are meant as a person, even if we are not. The grumpy face of the colleague, the neighbour who does not say hello again, the headache of the partner, the breaking copier, the dog excrement we have stepped in, the computer virus, the electronic mailbox full of spam mails, the bad grade in the math test of the son—all these things and many more we take as personally as possible. Either by feeling personally attacked, offended, or disrespected by them, or by blaming ourselves for them. So throughout the day, we will always find opportunities to get upset and stressed out.

Taking everything too personally

■ **Deficit Thinking**

This is a common variant of "view of the negative", which consists in focusing one's thoughts one-sidedly on one's own weaknesses, deficits, and past failures. Of course, it is necessary to deal with one's own weaknesses. But if this is done too one-sidedly without also looking at one's own strengths and successes, then this undermines our self-confidence, which we need in order to be able to face the demands calmly and confidently.

Overemphasize weaknesses and deficiencies

So far for the description of common stress aggravating thinking patterns. In the second part of this book, under the heading "Mental Stress Competence", we will turn to the question of what stress-reducing, beneficial thinking consists of and how it can be developed (▶ Chap. 7).

Stimulating Self-reflection: Stress Aggravating Thought Patterns

Please take a moment to examine which of the five stress aggravating thought patterns described above are more pronounced and which are less pronounced in your brain.

	Rather strongly pronounced	Rather low pronounced
"No way!" thinking		
View of the negative		
Negative consequences thinking		
Personalize		
Deficit thinking		

4.3 Five Stress Amplifiers and What Is Behind Them

"Must" thinking: desires are set in absolute terms

Whereas the previous section dealt with thought patterns that exacerbate stress, the following section will focus on internal setpoints that exacerbate stress. This refers to personal motives and goals, as well as internalized norms, which represent the internal yardstick against which we measure the personal significance of everyday situations and requirements (▶ Sect. 4.1). Characteristic of stress-intensifying set points is a "must" thinking. Motives, goals, or internalized norms are elevated to absolute demands, the fulfillment of which is seen as absolutely necessary for one's own well-being and self-esteem. Personal stress amplifiers ultimately consist of an exaggeration of inherently normal human motives. I will introduce five common personal stress amplifiers to you in the following.

▪ Be Perfect!

Desire for success

In the background of this stress amplifier is the achievement motive, the desire for success and self-affirmation through good performance. Those who are performance-motivated want to do something well, better or—best of all—best. If, however, this motive becomes overpowering and is raised to an absolute demand, then it is combined with a pronounced susceptibility to stress, especially towards those situations in which failure and one's own mistakes are possible or threatening. Perfectionist performance behaviour is an attempt to avoid such situations at all costs. The problem here is not one of wanting to improve or striving for peak performance. There are also, of course, areas of work in which the highest degree of accuracy and perfection are required. It becomes problematic when the perfectionist striving for performance is carried into all areas of life and transferred to any professional task or private activity. Sooner or later, this inevitably leads to excessive demands on oneself and finally to exhaustion. It often becomes particularly problematic when the achievement motive is linked to the commitment motive, that is when perfect achievements serve not only to confirm oneself but also to gain emotional affection from others. Such a constellation is often present in work addiction. This will be discussed further below.

■ **Be Popular!**

In the background of this stress amplifier is the binding motive, the desire to belong, to be accepted and loved. If this motive becomes overpowering and is raised to an absolute demand, then it is combined with a pronounced susceptibility to stress, especially in situations in which criticism and rejection by others are possible or threatened. It is also experienced as particularly stressful when one has to represent one's own interests, set limits and disappoint others, or when there are conflicts, differences of opinion, and the like with others. Such situations must be avoided or defused at all costs. This is attempted by putting one's own interests aside and trying to please literally everyone. Even an excessive willingness to help is sometimes in the service of the "Be popular!" booster. Certainly there are always situations in which it is necessary or appropriate to compromise, to give in, and to help others. The problem here again lies in overdoing it, in "too much of a good thing," which in the long run leads to self-overload and burnout.

Desire to be liked by all

■ **Be Independent!**

In the background of this stress amplifier is the autonomy motive, the desire for personal independence and self-determination. If this motive becomes overpowering and is raised to an absolute demand, then it is combined with a pronounced susceptibility to stress, especially in situations in which dependence on others, one's own need for help and weaknesses are experienced or threatened. People with a strong desire for autonomy therefore prefer to carry out their

Desire to be independent

tasks alone and deal with difficulties, worries, and anxieties on their own. They find it difficult to delegate, to work in a team, to ask others for help or support, and to confide in others. They try to maintain an image of strength and independence towards themselves and others at all costs. It is obvious that such behaviour can easily lead to self-exhaustion in the longer term.

Not allowed to show weaknesses

What exacerbates stress here is not the striving for independence, which is healthy in itself, but once again its one-sided exaggeration, which does not allow people to lean on others and let themselves be helped.

■ Keep Control!

Desire to remain in control

In the background of this stress amplifier is the control motive, the desire for security in and control over one's own life. If this motive becomes overpowering and is raised to an absolute demand, then it is combined with a pronounced susceptibility to stress, especially in situations in which loss of control, wrong decisions, and risks are possible or threatening. In order to avoid such situations, people with a strong desire for control try to have everything under their own control as much as possible. They also find it difficult to delegate. They tend to worry constantly about possible risks and dangers, and it takes them a lot of time and energy to make decisions for fear of overlooking possible risks. Thus, this stress amplifier can also promote self-overload and burnout in the longer term, as one hundred percent certainty and control cannot be achieved. Especially in times of increasing uncertainty, the striving for security needs to be balanced by the courage to take calculated risks, by letting go and by trust.

■ Hang in There!

Want to persevere

In the background of this stress amplifier is the central striving for pleasure and avoidance of displeasure, which here, however, is not too strongly pronounced, as is the case with other stress amplifiers, but on the contrary is too strongly suppressed. One is too hard on oneself. In the pursuit of goals, perseverance and gritting one's teeth are considered the highest maxims. This is also an attempt to avoid a confrontation with one's own limits, with excessive demands and failure. This can lead to not allowing oneself any breaks, to ignoring or denying signals of one's own need for rest, to holding on to unrealistic goals or unsolvable tasks for too long, thus driving oneself into exhaustion in the long run. Of course, it is an important, even necessary, skill to be able to overcome the wish for instant pleasure and to be able to face unpleasant tasks and leave one's comfort zone in the pursuit of goals. What is problematic here is again the exaggeration, a "too much of a good thing" that does not allow one to rest once in a while and to avoid unpleasant things or to allow the abandonment of a project or goal.

So much for the description of the five common personal stress amplifiers. Since they are based on common human motives, each of us carries each of these stressors to a greater or lesser degree. You can use the checklist in ▶ Sect. 4.6 at the end of this chapter to find out what your personal stress intensifiers are. In the second part of this book (▶ Sect. 7.4), we will look at how to reduce personal stressors.

The extent to which the five stress amplifiers or the motives behind them are individually pronounced is the result of the experiences gained in the course of one's biography. For example, someone who has had the experience from an early age that as soon as he articulates his own interests to others, for example to his parents, he is punished with withdrawal of love, will find the connection motive ("Be popular!") very important in adulthood. Those who had to make the experience at an early age that they cannot rely on other people will have the control motive ("Keep control!") and possibly also the autonomy motive ("Be independent!") strongly developed in adulthood. In adulthood, these biographically developed motive characteristics then shape the personal lens through which a wide variety of everyday situations are perceived as personal threats and, as a result, the biological stress program is triggered. At the end of this chapter, I would like to illustrate this in more detail using two examples.

4.4 **Perfectionist Control Ambitions**

The central theme here is control. The thoughts and behaviour of the affected people are dominated by the strong desire to have everything in their environment under their own control. These exaggerated ambitions of control show themselves, for example, in:

Want to control everything

- **Low tolerance for mistakes:** Mistakes (especially your own) must be avoided at all costs, are not tolerable as they indicate a possible loss of control.
- **Inability to delegate:** In order to maintain control, these people prefer to do everything themselves, taking care of anything and everything themselves. They are poor team workers, especially when the pressure is on. While they themselves are reluctant to delegate, they are the ones most likely to have new tasks or additional assignments delegated to them. This does not only refer to the field of work, but also, for example, to voluntary activities, work in associations, etc.

4

- **Impatience, irritability, irritability when things go wrong:** For these people, it is a disaster when things (or people) do not go or work the way they should. Disruptions also mean loss of control.
- **Suppression of relaxation needs:** The permanent effort to control goes hand in hand with a lack of awareness of one's own need to relax. Relaxation is difficult in the first place, because it means giving up control and letting go.

Lack of confidence

At the bottom of the soul, in most cases, lurks a fundamental, existential fear. There is a lack of fundamental trust in the orderliness and reliability of the world and of other people. The biographical background often includes experiences with less stable, fragile relationships with primary caregivers or with less reliable, unpredictable, erratic behaviour of caregivers. "If I don't control everything myself, keep it under control, chaos will break out". This worldview finds itself confirmed over and over again—like a self-fulfilling prophecy. The more these people pull everything to themselves, the more dependent the others become. Mistakes and wrong decisions actually become more frequent—a self-reinforcing vicious circle that is further accelerated by the fact that their tireless efforts receive praise and recognition. That's "someone who really puts in the work, who takes care of the last little things", is the appreciative comment from superiors and co-workers.

If the control fails ...

If this constant effort to control is already draining energy reserves, the situation becomes completely critical, not infrequently life-threatening, when these people are confronted with an objectively uncontrollable situation, for example, when restructuring is carried out in a company over a longer period of time over which they have no influence, when redundancies are imminent, or even when everyday work is determined by constantly changing demands or specifications. Such situations stimulate control ambitions. Those concerned react with intensified, undosed performance behaviour in order to regain control. With their aloof willingness to spend they eventually bring themselves into exhaustion crises, which they themselves, however, cannot adequately perceive.

4.5 Addiction to Work

Compulsion to work all the time

The term work addiction refers to the incessant urge or compulsion to constantly work or to constantly think about work. The observable behaviour of a work addict shows a great overlap with the behaviour of a person with perfectionistic control ambitions. However, the internal dynamics are different here. Whereas in the latter case, the striving for control also extends to areas of life outside of work, to family life, and hobbies, the thoughts and actions of the work addict are narrowed down solely to work.

The phenomenon cannot be grasped quantitatively, but only qualitatively. From how many hours of daily working time does a work addiction exist? There is no clear answer to this question. Work addicts do work long hours (but not necessarily effectively), but not everyone who works a lot or hard is a work addict. Work addicts do not just work a lot, they gain their self-worth and identity solely through work and achievement.

Characteristics of work addiction are the typical signs of addiction:

- **Denial and trivialization of** the addiction and its consequences. The workaholic trivializes, he becomes dishonest with himself and others, looks for excuses, works secretly under certain circumstances. Some trivialize or flirt with their problem by calling themselves a "workaholic".
- **Compulsivity**, which includes the inability to relax and the tendency to think about leisure during work and then—mediated by a guilty conscience—about work during leisure. Thinking is increasingly dominated by the drug "work".
- **Stockpiling**, dose increase and withdrawal symptoms: A completed job, a professional success cannot be enjoyed. New plans are always made, projects are designed, sometimes the completion of a job is delayed so that the work does not run out. More and more overtime is voluntarily worked, work is taken home, the bedroom is converted into an office, work is also taken on holiday, sometimes disguised as leisure reading. When those affected are forced not to work for once, they develop real withdrawal symptoms. They become restless, nervous, and irritable.
- **(Auto-)destructiveness**: Like any addiction, work addiction is accompanied by self-destruction and ruthless destruction of social relationships. The children are only in the way, spouses, who often show understanding for a long time in the sense of co-dependency, and pity the workaholic because of his workload, finally turn away unnerved. Broken families are regularly part of the full picture of work addiction.
- **Multiple addictions**: Secondary addictions often develop alongside the primary work addiction. Often, it is the excessive use of alcohol or medication to unwind. The secondary addiction is sometimes also used to justify or downplay the primary work addiction.

There is no fixed dividing line between normal and addictive work behaviour; the transitions are fluid. Some authors portray work addiction as an exaggeration of the normal, desired lifestyle in the modern working society, in which work is the centre of one's life and identity.

> Work determines self-worth

> Addiction to work is an addiction

Search for recognition

■ **Background: What Drives the Workaholic?**

As with all addictions, at the bottom of the soul you often find a longing. A **longing for recognition**, for being accepted as one is, for love. The work addict has learned that he gets recognition for performance. An experience that can be deeply rooted in childhood. And so he tries to satisfy his longing through achievement. But the recognition he receives for his performance cannot really satisfy his longing. What he was denied as a child, and what he unconsciously longs for as an adult, unconditional acceptance and being loved, this need ultimately remains unfulfilled. This leads to the misleading conclusion that the need is not yet satisfied only because not enough has been done. The urge for more and more work and achievement becomes life-determining.

Fear of failure

■ **Unstable Self-confidence and Fear of Failure**

What the workaholic lacks is a fundamental confidence in himself. If the person concerned has already had the experience at an early age that, for example, his school achievements are not sufficient to achieve the longed-for recognition on the part of his parents, the gnawing chronic feeling of not being good enough develops. In some cases, this feeling contributes to massive work inhibition. The individual works excessive hours, that is stays late at work, but avoids starting the important tasks, puts them off, gets distracted—for fear of failing. Feelings of guilt develop, driving him to work even longer.

Work as escape

■ **Escape from Inner Emptiness, from Personal Problems**

For many people, throwing themselves into work is also a tried and tested means, because it is socially accepted, of avoiding conflicts in the partnership or family or of covering up feelings of inner emptiness. Work degenerates into a drug that seems to help overcome deficits in experience and family problems. Even if escape is not always the primary driving force behind work addiction, in the course of time a vicious circle of long working hours, resulting family disputes, disappointments, reproaches, and increasing feelings of alienation develops in most people, which they try to avoid by working even more.

4.6 Checklist: Personal Stress Amplifiers

The following list contains a number of common stress aggravating thoughts (◼ Fig. 4.2). Please check how familiar you are with these thoughts (◼ Fig. 4.3).

Checklist: Stress aggravating thoughts				
How much do you agree with the following statements?				
	fully true	fairly true	Somewhat true	Does not apply
1. I prefer to do everything myself.	3	2	1	0
2. Giving up is never an option for me.	3	2	1	0
3. It's terrible when something doesn't go the way I want or planned.	3	2	1	0
4. I have to persevere at all costs.	3	2	1	0
5. If I really put my mind to it, I'll make it.	3	2	1	0
6. It's not acceptable if I don't get a job done or I don't meet a deadline.	3	2	1	0
7. I have to take the pressure (anxiety, pain, etc.) no matter what.	3	2	1	0
8. I always have to be there for my business.	3	2	1	0
9. You have to be really tough on yourself.	3	2	1	0
10. It's important that I have everything under control.	3	2	1	0
11. I don't want to disappoint the others.	3	2	1	0
12. There is nothing worse than making mistakes.	3	2	1	0
13. I have to be 100% reliable.	3	2	1	0
14. It is terrible when others are angry with me.	3	2	1	0
15. Strong people don't need help.	3	2	1	0
16. I want to get along with everyone.	3	2	1	0
17. It is terrible when others criticize me.	3	2	1	0
18. If I rely on others, I am abandoned.	3	2	1	0
19. It is important that everyone likes me.	3	2	1	0
20. When I make decisions, I have to be 100% sure.	3	2	1	0
21. I have to constantly think about what all might happen.	3	2	1	0
22. I without me it dose not work.	3	2	1	0
23. I always have to do everything right.	3	2	1	0
24. It's terrible to be dependent on others.	3	2	1	0
25. It's terrible when I don't know what's coming.	3	2	1	0

Fig. 4.2 Checklist: Stress aggravating thoughts

4

Personal stress amplifier profile

Evaluation of the checklist "Stress Aggravating Thoughts"

(1) Add the scores to thoughts 6, 8, 12, 13, and 23.

Value 1 = _____

(2) Add the scores to thoughts 11, 14, 16, 17, and 19.

Value 2 = _____

(3) Add the scores to thoughts 1, 15, 18, 22, and 24.

Value 3 = _____

(4) Add the scores to thoughts 3, 10, 20, 21, and 25.

Value 4 = _____

(5) Add the scores to thoughts 2, 4, 5, 7, and 9.

Value 5 = _____

(6) Transfer the calculated values 1 to 5 to the graph.

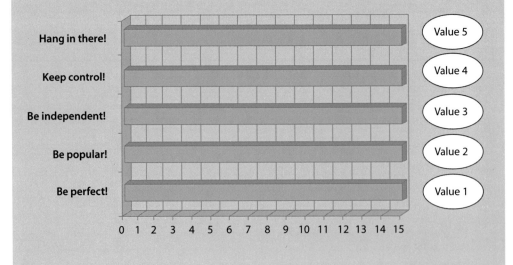

□ **Fig. 4.3** Personal stress intensifier profile

Coping with Stress

Contents

What Can We Do? The Three Pillars of Stress Competence at a Glance

Contents

© Springer-Verlag GmbH Germany, part of Springer Nature 2022
G. Kaluza, *Calm and Confident Under Stress*, https://doi.org/10.1007/978-3-662-64440-9_5

5

What is successful stress management?

What are the degrees of freedom and scope of action open to us for stress management? What possibilities do we have to deal with the demands of everyday life at work, in the family and in our leisure time in a more relaxed and confident manner and thus in a way that is beneficial to our health and well-being?

On the following pages, I will give you an initial overview of the three main starting points and the three main pillars of individual stress management. In doing so, I am assuming a broad understanding of stress management. What is meant here are not only all measures to get a grip on physical and mental stress reactions that have already occurred, but also all efforts to reduce stressful demands, to change them, to reduce them or to avoid them altogether, as well as to review and change one's own attitudes and evaluations.

To counter a possible misunderstanding from the outset, which I often encounter when it comes to the topic of "stress management": the goal of stress management is not to live a life that is as low in demands as possible. It is not about propagating a life in which one avoids as much effort as possible, "taking it easy" on an energetic zero line through life, so to speak. Successful stress management rather aims at a healthy handling of external and self-imposed demands. It is about using one's own energy to deal with the demands of everyday life in a way that promotes health and well-being.

Balance of tension and relaxation

It is of crucial importance that we find a balance between phases of tension, commitment, and engagement on the one hand, which are repeatedly replaced by phases of relaxation, recuperation, and distancing from the demands on the other. The longer and the harder I commit myself to a cause, the longer and more intensive the subsequent time for relaxation and recuperation must be.

No patent remedies

It is also not my intention to provide you with simple advice and patent remedies. Because they do not really exist. Just as the development of stress is individual, a promising stress management strategy must also be individual and tailor-made. I will point out different ways. Your task will be to pick out what you can use to cope with your own personal stressors at work and in everyday life.

Before you read on, I would first ask you to think about your own stress management strategies that you have already used (▶ Box 5.1).

Box 5.1: To Get Started: My Stress Management Skills
What stress management options do you already use yourself? What do you already do? Which strategies have you had good experiences with so far? What helps you to cope with your everyday demands?

Take some time to answer these questions in order to become aware of your own existing competences. If you wish, write down your answers. This will give you an initial collection of successful stress management strategies that you can add to as you read this book.

Let us now try to sort out the different strategies of stress management and put them in order. The three-part stress model (▶ Chap. 1, ◘ Fig. 1.1) can help us to do this. With this model in mind, we can distinguish three main starting points and three main pillars of individual stress competence (◘ Fig. 5.1).

■ **Starting Point Stressors**
The goal here is to prevent stress from arising in the first place. On the one hand, we can achieve this by influencing the external demands, that is the stressors in the professional and private spheres, changing them and, as far as possible, reducing or eliminating them altogether. On the other hand, we can also prevent the development of stress by developing our own—professional and social—skills for coping with demands. Stress management experts also speak of **instrumental stress management** or **instrumental stress competence**.

Instrumental stress competence

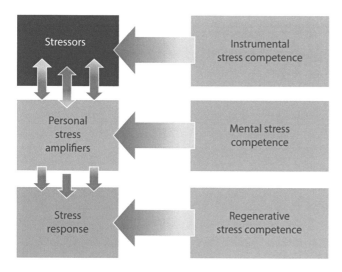

◘ **Fig. 5.1** The three pillars of stress competence

Mental stress competence

■ **Starting Point Personal Stress Amplifiers**

This involves becoming self-critically aware of one's own stress-producing or stress-exacerbating attitudes, evaluations, and mental patterns, gradually changing them and replacing them with beneficial thoughts and attitudes. In this case, experts also speak of **mental stress management** or **mental stress competence.**

Regenerative stress competence

■ **Starting Point Stress Reactions**

This is about releasing existing physical tension, dampening inner restlessness and nervousness, and maintaining one's own resistance to stress in the longer term. It is about relaxation and recovery. The expert term for this is: **regenerative stress management** or **regenerative stress competence**.

Preventing the development of stress

5.1 Instrumental Stress Management: Making Everyday Life Less Stressful

Instrumental stress management ultimately aims at preventing the development of stress. To this end, one can start with the stressors with the aim of reducing or completely eliminating them, for example, by reorganizing the workplace, by changing work processes, by organizing assistance, etc. Or one starts with oneself with the aim of further developing one's own competences which are necessary to cope with the demands. Instrumental stress management can be reactive in response to concrete, current stress situations and can also be proactive in reducing or eliminating future stress (▶ Box 5.2).

> **Box 5.2: Examples of Instrumental Stress Management**
> ▬ Enhance professional competencies (information, training, peer exchange).
> ▬ Organizational improvements (distribution of tasks, workflow planning, filing systems, etc.).
> ▬ Self-management: optimize personal work organization (define personal/professional priorities, realistic time planning, delegation).
> ▬ Develop social-communicative skills (set boundaries for others, say "no", "without me", "not now" more often, say something positive, understand others, talk things out, have clarifying conversations).
> ▬ Seek support (get help, ask for support, network).
> ▬ Develop problem-solving skills.

Of course, not all burdens can be reduced in this way. However, do not dismiss these possibilities too quickly. Often it is not so much objective, unchangeable circumstances as one's own attitudes about oneself and others that stand in the way of reducing burdens. Those who consider themselves indispensable will obviously have difficulty delegating tasks. Someone who always wants to do everything 150% will hardly be able to set clear priorities. Those who always want to please everyone and not disappoint anyone will hardly ever be able to say "no".

Instrumental stress management requires a level of expertise sufficient to meet the respective requirements. In this respect, professional qualification represents an important instrumental strategy for stress management. However, professional competence alone is often not sufficient. Instrumental stress management also requires social-communicative skills and **self-management skills** as the ability to act in a self-directed and goal-oriented manner.

We will discuss instrumental stress management strategies in detail in ▶ Chap. 6.

5.2 Mental Stress Management: Developing Supportive Attitudes and Evaluations

Mental statements on stressful events often run almost automatically and have become so second nature to us that they appear to us as the only possible self-evident "truth". The insight that our own evaluation is only one—subjective—possibility among several how things can be viewed is not easy. For this insight also means, under certain circumstances, saying goodbye to the maxims of life that we have grown fond of, as well as to clear assignments of guilt and habitual comfortable patterns of thought.

Changing your own evaluation

Mental stress management aims to change stress-producing or stress-exacerbating personal motives, attitudes, and evaluations, that is personal stress amplifiers. The aim of mental stress management strategies is to make people aware of these, to reflect critically on them and to transform them into stress-reducing, beneficial attitudes, and evaluations (▶ Box 5.3).

Box 5.3: Examples of Mental Stress Management
- Critically examine perfectionist performance expectations and learn to accept one's own performance limits.
- See difficulties not as a threat but as a challenge.

5

> — Identify less personally with everyday tasks, maintain more inner distance.
> — Not to get lost in the everyday petty wars, to keep an eye on the "essentials", on what is really important to me.
> — Becoming aware of what is positive, enjoyable, successful and feeling gratitude for it.
> — Do not get stuck on unpleasant feelings of hurt or anger, but learn to let them go and forgive.
> — Have less fixed ideas and expectations of others, accept reality.
> — Take yourself less important, get rid of false pride and learn "humility".

Mental stress management strategies are discussed in detail in ▶ Chap. 7.

5.3 Regenerative Stress Management: Relax and Recover

Alleviate the effects of stress

Physical and mental stress reactions can never be completely avoided. We have already repeatedly emphasized in the previous chapters that this would not make sense and would not be desirable. Successful stress management therefore always includes strategies to relieve existing physical tension and to dampen inner restlessness and nervousness with the aim of alleviating negative stress consequences in the long term, as well as strategies that serve to maintain one's own resistance to stress and to build up new energies (▶ Box 5.4).

> **Box 5.4: Examples of Regenerative Stress Management**
> — Regular practice of a relaxation technique,
> — Regular exercise,
> — A healthy, varied diet,
> — Maintaining extra-occupational social contacts,
> — Regular compensation through hobbies and leisure activities,
> — Learn to enjoy the little things in everyday life,
> — Adequate sleep.

We will get to know possibilities of regenerative stress management in detail in ▶ Chap. 8.

5.4 Flexibility as a Goal: Finding Your Own Way

What characterizes successful stress management in the long term? There is no generally valid answer to this question. There are no patent remedies. Since stress is individual, it is important that you, dear readers, find your own, very personal way. How can you do that?

Of elementary importance here is first of all to be able to distinguish between those stressful situations whose occurrence and course one can influence oneself, and those stressful situations over which one cannot exert any direct influence. The German-American theologian and philosopher Reinhard Niebuhr (1892–1971) addresses precisely this distinction in his "Serenity Prayer", which has achieved great popularity as the motto of Alcoholics Anonymous:

> » God grant me the serenity to accept the things I cannot change, the courage to change the things I can, and the wisdom to discern one from the other.

Successful stress management is largely based on this wisdom Niebuhr speaks of. It enables us to react flexibly and appropriately to the situation. It frees us from the passive victim role and opens up inner freedom, which is the foundation of any successful long-term stress management. This inner freedom also includes—what is sometimes overlooked—the freedom to decide for ourselves if, when and how we actually change a situation we can influence. We do not necessarily have to approach every controllable situation instrumentally. We can also choose to accept the situation as it is and change our attitude towards it. Whether it is worth it to us is a matter of our free choice. Even in situations whose occurrence and course we cannot influence by our own behaviour, we are not merely helpless victims. Our freedom here lies in choosing our own attitude to the situation in question and in becoming active in the sense of regenerative stress management in order to limit or completely prevent negative stress consequences.

However, if this inner freedom is not to remain just a theoretical possibility, but if we actually want to choose freely and flexibly how to deal with a stressful situation, then this requires that we also have the necessary skills to do so. Effective stress management is therefore based on a repertoire of stress management skills that is as broad as possible and encompasses all three of the pillars described. It includes instrumental as well as mental and regenerative strategies.

It is important here to avoid one-sidedness and to achieve a balance between the three pillars of stress competence (◘ Fig. 5.2). "Too much of a good thing" ultimately turns

Can I change anything?

Is it worth it to me?

Stress management requires skills

"Too much of a good thing": avoid one-sidedness

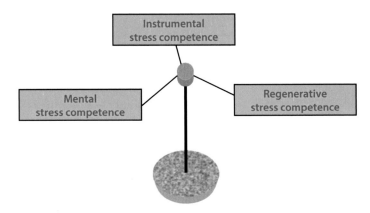

◻ Fig. 5.2   Stress competence in balance

5

into a negative in the field of stress management as well. Those who exclusively and constantly strive for active control of demands without also making use of opportunities for distraction, relaxation, and problem distancing will ultimately fruitlessly "sink their teeth" into "problems" and wear themselves out in the process. Whoever—conversely—tries to cope with stress exclusively through regenerative measures such as sports and relaxation exercises, for example, without also actively dealing with the respective demands in an instrumental or mental way, is virtually fleeing reality and is literally trying to run away from demands and difficulties, ultimately in vain.

Expand one's coping repertoire

If you would like to further develop your personal stress competence, you should therefore direct your attention primarily to those areas that are less developed in your current coping repertoire. In order to avoid too one-sided a development of your personal stress competence and to expand your scope of action, you should therefore not proceed according to the "more of the same" principle, but rather try out and integrate such strategies that you have not practiced so far, or have practiced only rarely. If you have so far tried to cope with stress at work and in everyday life mainly in a regenerative way, for example, through relaxation, distraction, and compensation, you should focus on strategies of instrumental and mental stress management. And vice versa: those who have so far mainly relied on active strategies in the sense of instrumental stress management when dealing with stress, for example, seeking support, delegation, setting limits, and good time management, should give priority to dealing with mental and especially regenerative strategies.

In the following chapters, you will receive suggestions for all three pillars of individual stress competence. Pick out what promises the greatest benefit in terms of expanding your personal stress competence.

Stimulus for Self-reflection: My Personal Stress Competence
— What are my strengths in stress management?
— Which of the three pillars of stress competence are strong in me, and which are less strong?
— What do I want to learn in order to expand my personal stress competence? Where do I see a need for personal development?

Actively Meeting Demands: Instrumental Stress Competence

Contents

© Springer-Verlag GmbH Germany, part of Springer Nature 2022
G. Kaluza, *Calm and Confident Under Stress*, https://doi.org/10.1007/978-3-662-64440-9_6

This chapter deals with ways of instrumental stress management, that is reducing stressors in work and everyday life as far as possible or changing them in such a way that less stress occurs. It is also about organizing one's own everyday life in such a way that unnecessary stress does not occur in the first place.

Even if it sometimes seems like it: we are not completely helpless in the face of the stressors in our everyday lives. We have possibilities for action. Of course, not all stressors can be eliminated, and that would not be sensible or desirable. But we can, at least to a certain extent, influence which demands we want to face and which we do not. And we can work on ourselves, expand our competencies in order to be able to meet current and future demands more easily and with less stress. It is therefore important to recognize our own room for manoeuvre and to exploit it as far as possible.

Identify possible courses of action

Instrumental stress competence essentially consists of four components (◨ Fig. 6.1):

1. Professional competences and expertise to cope with the performance requirements,
2. Social skills to build and maintain a supportive social network,
3. The competence to assert oneself, that is to represent one's own interests appropriately and to set limits, and
4. Self-management competence as the ability to independently control one's life according to self-defined goals.

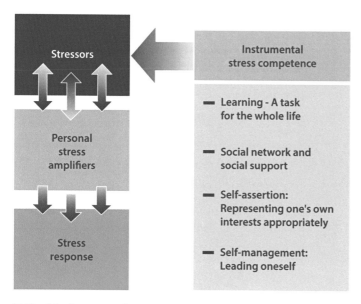

◨ **Fig. 6.1** Instrumental stress competence

These components of instrumental stress competence and their importance for successful stress management will be discussed in the following sections of this chapter.

6.1 Learning: A Lifelong Task

Willingness to learn

In our time of rapid technological change, the half-life of knowledge is getting shorter and shorter. What one has learned in school, training or studies is usually no longer sufficient for a whole professional life. This applies not only to job-specific knowledge in the narrower sense, but also, for example, to language skills, which are becoming increasingly important in internationally active companies, as well as the competent use of modern communication media and dealing with the flood of information with which we are confronted every day. In order to protect ourselves effectively and in the long term against gradual loss of competence, increasing excessive demands, and premature wear and tear, a willingness to engage in lifelong learning is therefore essential.

Do you sometimes feel like the woodsman (▶ Box 6.1)? Have you also neglected to sharpen your tools regularly in the course of your professional life? As explained in the first part of this book, stress always arises when we are confronted with demands that we consider important to meet, but at the same time we are uncertain whether our abilities will be sufficient to do so. The fear of not being able to meet the expectations placed on us, of no longer being able to cope with the pressure of competition, also the fear that our own insecurities could be noticed by others, possibly even used against us—all this can trigger a strong experience of stress.

> **Box 6.1: Story of the Woodsman**
> This is the story of the woodsman who, full of verve, cuts down trees with a saw. Initially, he makes quick progress. But as time goes by, his performance decreases, causing the man to work even harder. But no matter how hard he tries, his pace decreases even more. Sweating and grumbling, he works away without getting much closer to his goal. Then a walker passes by, and, after watching the workman for some time, asks him, "Good man, wouldn't it be more useful if you sharpened the saw first?" To this the workman angrily replies, "No, I really have no time for that now. I have to saw, saw, saw ..." (Source: unknown)

It is quite clear: only those who regularly sharpen their saw, that is keep their professional knowledge and skills up to date, will be able to hold their own in professional life with success and without unnecessary stress in the longer term. And the earlier you start, the less effort is ultimately required for this.

"Sharpening His Saw"

If you are suffering from a high level of stress in your everyday professional life, then you should seriously ask yourself whether your experience of stress might not be caused, at least in part, by the fact that in your current professional position you are confronted with demands that you have not been trained to cope with, or have been trained insufficiently to cope with (► Box 6.2).

> **Box 6.2: Self-reflection: Is Your Saw Still Sharp?**
> — What are the main professional requirements you need to meet in your current professional position (or in a position you aspire to)?
> — Where do you see your current professional strengths and competencies?
> — Where is there a need for development? What would you like to learn?

"I don't have time for this. I have more important things to do ...". This is how many people think and act—much like the woodsman in our story—when it comes to their own continuing education and training. It is obvious that this is an extremely short-sighted view. It is also clear that developing your own professional skills takes time. For this, the necessary time freedoms must be found and defended against disruptions. Clear priorities and good time management can be helpful here (we will look at this in more detail in later sections of this chapter). Initiative and commitment on the part of the individual are just as important here as support from superiors and employers.

Make time for training

Continuing professional development should not only take place reactively to new requirements that have already been set, but should also be pursued proactively. This means that one should continuously inform oneself about innovations and trends that are relevant for one's own profession or the wider professional environment or could become interesting in the future.

Stay up to date

The opportunities offered for further professional qualification are extremely diverse. The range extends from specialist journals to specialist conferences, seminars, and workshops to part-time advanced training courses. The Internet also offers

Take advantage of offers

up to date information portals, newsletters, and forums for the exchange of information on almost every specialist topic. Supervision and coaching also offer helpful opportunities for further professional qualification, especially when it comes to transferring acquired knowledge into everyday professional practice and overcoming difficulties that arise in the process.

Learning from others

Finally, everyday professional life itself, the exchange with colleagues, customers, or competitors, offers repeated opportunities to update one's knowledge. The most important thing here is to maintain one's curiosity and inquisitiveness and not be afraid to learn from others. Rather than highlighting your own expertise and knowledge, this means not being afraid to ask questions, admitting that you do not know something, listening and encouraging others to share their knowledge. Ultimately, it is about seeing oneself less as a "knower" and more as a "learner".

6.2 Maintaining Networks: Social Relationships as a Stress Buffer

Social ties protect health

Interpersonal contacts are not only a frequent source of stressful experiences, but also a very important resource in dealing with stress. It is one of the best established findings of health psychology research: a well-established social network protects health. Satisfying contacts with other people can make it easier to cope with stress and protect us from the harmful effects of stress. They reduce feelings of loneliness and excessive demands, allow pain to be forgotten and anger to dissipate.

For children, reliable social ties are the most important prerequisite for healthy physical and mental development. As early as the 1950s, the very well-known studies by the developmental psychologist Rene Spitz (1887–1974) on children in hospitals and orphanages showed what devastating effects a lack of human attention can have.

Social support at the workplace

Stable social ties are also an important protective health factor for adults. Scientific studies have repeatedly shown: people who feel well embedded socially have a relatively low risk of falling ill in stressful situations. On the other hand, people who say they do not have sufficiently satisfying social relationships suffer with above-average frequency from depression, psychosomatic illnesses, and weakened immune competence. In working life, too, social support and satisfying social contacts with colleagues and superiors play a decisive role not only for job satisfaction, performance, and willingness to perform, but also as effective protection against burning out.

Practical aids

In this context, the support and sustainment that we can experience through positive interpersonal contacts are extremely multifaceted. Through exchanges with others, we can receive important new information and advice that can help us solve problems. Other people can provide very practical support when, for example, one is overburdened with work or has a need in everyday life.

But not only that. Talking with others about one's own burdens can also bring relief and new courage. We can experience comfort and encouragement from others and experience that someone stands by us. Shared experiences of physical and emotional closeness, mutual acceptance, and trust form a real protective mantle against which the stressors of everyday life are buffered. Physical contact, tenderness, and sexuality lower the level of stress hormones and create a deep feeling of relaxation and well-being. To be perceived, acknowledged, and appreciated by others is essential for one's own self-esteem. Being with others also often makes it easier for us to switch off and "take our mind off things".

Emotional closeness

And we can have the equally positive experience of spiritual community, sharing with others views of life, values, and norms.

Spiritual community

The biological basis for the pain-relieving, anxiety-relieving, and stress-relieving effects of positive social relationships is probably to be seen in an increased release of the oxytocin known as the bonding hormone. Oxytocin is released not only during childbirth and breastfeeding in both mother and child, but whenever we feel securely attached in a positive social relationship—a social relationship in which we feel accepted as we are, in which we can let go and trust, in which we experience physical and emotional closeness. Via an increase in endogenous opioids, oxytocin leads to an increase in pain perception thresholds in such situations. In addition, it causes a decrease in heart rate, blood pressure, and cortisol concentration in the blood as well as an increased activity of the gastrointestinal tract, that is it has clear stress-reducing effects.

Social Network Analysis: Who Belongs to It?

The social network includes all persons with whom one has any kind of relationship. As a rule, these are close family members and relatives, neighbours, work colleagues, and friends. These can each serve different support functions: spouses and close friends can be particularly important for emotional support, neighbours for practical help and work colleagues for relevant information in solving problems.

It is important to become aware of the diversity of relationships in one's own social network and to learn to appreciate them. Every person has different sides and interests that can come into play in different relationships. With one person you like to fool

Valuing diversity in social relationships

around, with another you can have deep conversations, with the third you can work well together. You do not have to share all opinions and interests with everyone, and you should be careful not to project all relationship desires onto just one person (often that is your spouse). Your partner is not your colleague, your neighbour is not your friend, your colleague is not your neighbour, and yet each has an important meaning. Even friend is not friend. There are different forms of friendship, such as friends for common interests and hobbies, historical friends, for example, from school and university days, friendships between generations and finally the close friendships, the best friend.

Important: to be able to let yourself go

The average relationship network of a German adult comprises about 25 people, four to six each from family/relatives, neighbourhood, work, and leisure. About 50 % of the relationships from the social network are experienced as emotionally important and about two thirds as supportive. As you consider your own social network (▶ Box 6.3), please do not misunderstand these numbers as a standard to be met. Ultimately, it is not the number of network members that matters, but the quality of the relationships. For the stress-reducing effect of the social network, it is crucial that one can give oneself as one is in the relationship with others, that one feels accepted as the person one is, that one can let oneself go in the relationship.

Box 6.3: Observe and Reflect: My Social Network

The following exercise is designed to encourage you to think about your social network (◼ Fig. 6.2).

1. Write your name or "I" in a circle on the centre of as large a sheet of paper as possible. Divide the sheet into different areas that correspond to your areas of life: Family/relatives, work, neighbourhood, leisure/friends, etc.
2. Then, for each person in your social circle, draw a circle with the person's first letters or first name. By moving away from the "I" circle, you can represent the intensity of your relationship with that person: the closer the person's circle is to the "I" circle, the more intense the relationship. Different groups of people can also be represented by different coloured circles, for example, family members with yellow circles, relatives with blue circles, friends and acquaintances with red circles, neighbours with green circles, and so on.
3. Take a quiet look at your social network and pay special attention to the relationships that you experience as positive, supportive, or appreciative, with whom you feel comfortable. Mark these positive relationships with an exclamation mark next to each person's circle. The thicker the exclamation point, the more positive the relationship.

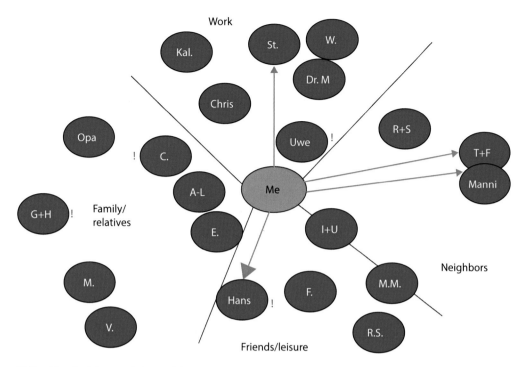

Fig. 6.2 Social network (example)

Maintaining the Social Network

» He who does not care for his nets need not be surprised at a lack of yield. (Old fishermen's wisdom)

In our open society, social networks have become fragile. Social relationships established through tradition are losing their binding force. The individual has to weave his or her own social network. The local mobility required in the modern world of work means that people may have to rebuild at least part of their everyday social network several times in their lives or maintain it over long distances. This is not only negative, but also holds the chance to develop richer, more open and needs-oriented social networks.

Everyone has to create his own social network

Critical life events (▶ Chap. 3), such as the death of a partner, divorce or separation, children moving out, etc., often lead to severe cuts in the social network. Those affected are then confronted with the difficult task of establishing new social contacts in a phase of great emotional stress.

Social networks rarely develop by themselves. Building and maintaining them usually take a lot of effort, are always associated with disappointments, and require a high degree of

Relationship capability

social competence. What is meant here is the ability to relate. This is the ability to enter into and maintain positive relationships with other people. This means, for example:

— Respond to offers of contact from others,
— Send out signals of willingness to make contact yourself,
— Start and maintain a conversation,
— Adjust to different people,
— Showing interest in the other,
— Empathy, understanding the other,
— Listen,
— Inquire,
— Make and maintain eye contact,
— Say something positive, give compliments, express praise and appreciation.

Practical Tips for Maintaining the Social Network
What can you concretely do in everyday life to maintain your social network? Here are some practical tips collected by participants of an anti-stress seminar:

— Give someone your regards
— Inquiring about someone
— Seek advice
— Ask someone a small favour
— Tell something about yourself
— Keeping yourself available to others
— Build up regularity (e.g. every 3rd Wednesday of the month ...)
— Remember birthdays, anniversaries, etc.
— Note and search for occasions for contact
— Introduce yourself (to strangers)
— Have attractive business cards with you
— Addressing someone directly, being open and curious
— Praise, express appreciation
— Compliment
— Saying thank you
— Just send an e-mail/postcard/SMS (without cause)
— Use social networks on the Internet (Facebook, etc.)
— Share pleasant news
— Offer his help
— Show interest in others, inquire
— Listen

"Real friends are always there for each other" and other blockades

» Take people as they are, there are no others! (Konrad Adenauer, first Chancellor of the Federal Republic of Germany, 1876–1967)

Misconceptions and inflated expectations are often a barrier to building social relationships. "Good neighbours always help", "Good girlfriends meet several times a week", "A real friend understands everything". With such inadequate ideas of social bonds, disappointments are virtually pre-programmed. One feels lost and abandoned, even if other people are actually present, who, however, do not meet the high expectations and who often feel overwhelmed by this and, therefore, withdraw.

Excessive expectations

A wide variety of fears can also hinder the development and maintenance of social relationships. In addition to the fear of rejection and disappointment, the fear of dependence on other people plays a role here. One fears having to commit oneself to something, to show gratitude or to conform.

Fear of rejection or dependence

Some people go through their everyday life with generalized negative images about their fellow human beings. "The others don't understand me anyway, they have no interest in me, they reject me, they are much too egoistic anyway, they only care about themselves and think only of themselves...". Such images of others act like a self-fulfilling prophecy. They also serve to protect oneself. Those who are afraid of rejection can also protect themselves by claiming that others are not attractive anyway.

Negative images about others

Such unrealistic expectations, fears, and negative images are not mere fantasies. They are based on real earlier, often very early relationship experiences—experiences of rejection, loneliness, disappointment, and dependence. The problem is that these experiences are over-generalized and transferred unchecked and unconsciously to current relationships. This then leads to the fact that the previous negative relationship experiences are always repeated, confirmed, and solidified in the present. You do not give yourself a chance to have new more positive experiences with other people. If we become aware of our own patterns of expectations, fears, and images and also understand their biographical background, then these patterns lose at least part of their power. We are no longer completely at their mercy and inner spaces open up that we can use to have new experiences.

Reflect: Maintaining the Social Network
Take a moment to look at the sheet with your social network (❒ Fig. 6.2) and think about the people in your social network with whom you would like to renew or strengthen contact. Connect the circles with the names of these people to the "I" circle in the middle with an arrow.

6.3 Self-assertion: Representing One's Own Interests Appropriately

Representing one's own needs

In addition to maintaining positive interpersonal relationships, this is the second component of social competence: self-assertion. Asserting oneself, maintaining one's own boundaries, interests, and needs appropriately and representing them to others is an important and necessary protection to keep oneself from being overwhelmed and stressed.

Setting Boundaries: For Yourself and Others

Say no

Probably, the most important and at the same time most difficult point for many people is saying "no", that is rejecting the demands or requests of others. The effort to never disappoint others and to always want to please everyone usually hinders a self-protective "no". Realize that you are not solely responsible for fulfilling all the wishes and demands of others. You have a right to your "no"! The point here is to set clear boundaries with others. This also requires that you feel your own limits in the first place and that you accept that your own capacity to perform has limits that need to be respected. This is especially difficult for committed, performance-oriented and helpful people, but it is of extreme importance in order to prevent a creeping decline in performance and burnout. In the following, I will give some examples of how such boundaries can look in practice, which were compiled in a stress management seminar for branch managers of a savings bank.

Setting Boundaries (Examples)

- Divert telephone (call forwarding, answering machine),
- Put up a "Do Not Disturb" sign,
- set up fixed office hours,
- Set a time limit for meetings and stick to it,
- Use the recycle bin ("Delete" button),
- Limit e-mail flood, therefore check e-mails regularly, but at fixed times (not constantly),
- Disable e-mail notification feature,
- Say "no", "not now", "without me" more often,
- Switch mobile phone, Blackberry etc. off or on at fixed times,
- Block off times for private/family things.

> **Observing and Reflecting: Thinking "No"—SAYING "Yes"**
> Do you sometimes think "no" and then say "yes"? In order to make visible how often this happens to you in everyday life, try the following illustrative method: in the morning, put many 1-cent coins in your right jacket pocket. Whenever you say "yes" at work or at home during the day, although you mean "no", put a coin from your right pocket into your left pocket. When you check in the evening how many coins you have in your left pocket, ask yourself self-critically in which situations you could have said "no" without really serious disadvantages.

Seek Support and Hand Over Tasks

Along with setting boundaries, seeking support is part of any practice of healthy assertiveness. This may surprise those who mistakenly confuse assertiveness with lone wolfism and "lonely strength". Nor is it about supplicating, but about confidently expressing desires, making one's own demands, and, wherever possible, handing off and delegating tasks. Accepting support is particularly difficult for many people. Fear of rejection or obligation and the feeling that expressing a request is tantamount to an admission of personal weakness play a role here. Are you one of those people who would rather help others than be helped yourself? Give your fellow human beings the chance to help you too! This brings relief for you personally. And for those to whom you hand over tasks or ask for support, this often also means motivation, a sign of confidence, and the opportunity to develop further.

Let us support you!

However, it is also clear that those who hand over tasks to others and thus rely on others run the risk of possible disappointment. This cannot be completely ruled out, but it can be minimized through increasing experience with which tasks can be handed over to whom. It is also helpful, and ultimately necessary, to have the inner willingness to accept that others will approach tasks differently than you do and that the result will not be exactly the same as it would have been if you had done the task yourself. Even if this inner readiness and also the insight that one cannot do everything alone are present, the handing over of tasks often fails in practice because it costs more time at the beginning. Time to prepare the tasks, to give explanations and instructions. In day-to-day business, it is tempting to quickly complete the task yourself. However, this additional investment of time is necessary and sensible in

6

order to experience relief in the long term and to gain free-dom. If you never take the time to show your children how to make the bed, you will have to do this task yourself until the children leave the house (or even beyond). If you never take the time to explain to your colleagues or employees how to deal with a certain customer inquiry, you will just keep finding these inquiries on your own desk.

> **To Think Ahead: Getting Support**
> You do not have to do everything yourself. Consider for which tasks you can enlist the support of people in your environment (neighbours, friends, relatives, colleagues, employees, etc.) or whether you can delegate tasks to these people. Perhaps there are people in your environment who are literally waiting to get a chance from you. This brings relief for you personally. And for those whom you ask for support, this often also means a sign of confidence and the opportunity to develop further.

Express Anger Appropriately

Pent-up anger

Suppressed anger increases inner agitation and physical ten-sion. If the anger is pent up, it often comes to an explosion at some point. It then takes only a small occasion to bring the barrel to overflow. Such a sudden outburst of anger is then usually hardly understandable for fellow human beings and only creates new problems. In order to deal with feelings of anger in a healthy way, it is important to accept everyday anger, even about seemingly trivial things, and to express it as early as possible. The other person can then accept and understand the anger more easily without leading to a lasting upset. So take your anger seriously and give the other person a chance to understand your anger.

Forgiven

So that there is no misunderstanding here: this is not a plea for uninhibited and uncontrolled expression of one's anger, for this usually leads not only to further argument with the other person, who is now angry in turn at the way you are dealing with him. If you give vent to your anger in an uncontrolled way, it also often happens that you really get carried away. Instead of feeling relief, anger and tension become even stron-ger. Sometimes it is wiser to first process the anger "within", not just swallow it down, but consciously let go and forgive the other person—even if it sounds old-fashioned. And the good thing about it is that you thereby gain a piece of inner freedom. You are no longer the victim of your feelings of anger, but you have the decision whether and what you are angry about or not.

Assertiveness Can Be Learned
Please think about situations in which you would like to say "no" or ask someone else for something. Play through the situation in your mind beforehand. Think about the words you would like to use. Imagine the reaction of others and think about how you will respond. At the next opportunity, put your "no" or your "please" or your "I want" into action. To begin with, choose simple situations with people who do not mean that much to you and with whom the contact is not so close, possibly even complete strangers, e.g. in a restaurant, in the canteen, in a train compartment, at the department store checkout.

If you ever lose your courage, then make yourself clear: self-assertion does not mean ruthlessness towards others. Rather, it means expressing your own wishes, needs, and feelings clearly and unambiguously in such a way that they can be accepted and understood by others. In this sense, assertiveness can also contribute to making relationships with other people more open and trusting, and thus to deepening them.

Self-assertion does not mean ruthlessness

6.4 Self-management: Managing Yourself

» Life can only be understood by looking backwards, but only lived by looking forwards. (Sören Kierkegaard, Danish philosopher, 1813–1851)

As important as adequate professional and good social skills are for dealing calmly and confidently with stress at work and in everyday life, self-management is even more important. In a way, this is the supreme discipline of instrumental stress management. It is about the ability to align one's own life with one's own professional and personal goals and to keep it in balance. In times of increasing external uncertainty, it is crucial that individuals find security and stability within themselves. Self-management essentially involves the ability to make decisions and the courage to set priorities. Both are indispensable in order not to drown in the abundance of possibilities that modern multi-option societies have in store for us and to protect ourselves from (self-)overload, constant time pressure and ultimately from burning out. Self-management also means: acting instead of reacting, following your own compass instead of always responding to external demands and pressures.

Follow the inner compass

6

Self-management starts with the simple realization, **"You can't do it all!"**—at least not all at once. This realization asks us to pause to rethink our own perspective on life and clarify our own values and goals. What is really important to me? What am I doing all this for? Where do I want to go? These are the questions we put to ourselves and to which we must find our own personal answers. Dealing with these fundamental questions is of course not a one-time thing, found answers are rarely valid for all times. Also, different phases of life often have different goals and priorities. It is therefore a process of self-discovery, a path on which one embarks—again and again—and in the course of which one's own compass gradually emerges.

What Really Counts: Clarifying Values and Goals

» He who has a wherefore to live, endures almost every how. (Friedrich W. Nietzsche, philosopher, 1844-1900)

Goals create meaning

Personal values and goals give meaning to one's own life. The conviction and the feeling of the meaningfulness of one's own life represent a significant health protection factor, because they help to actively cope with stress or to bear it more easily. This is shown, for example, by the very well-known studies of the Israeli stress researcher Aaron Antonovsky. In the early 1970s, Antonovsky conducted a study in Israel of women born between 1914 and 1923. The women studied had been born in Central Europe and some had been imprisoned in a concentration camp. Despite the almost unimaginable horror of the concentration camp, despite the subsequent odyssey that often lasted for years, and finally the emigration to Israel, where they then experienced three wars against the neighbouring Arab states, despite all these extremely stressful life experiences, about one third of the women were in a good state of mental and physical health at the time of the study.

Sense as a health protection factor

According to Antonovsky's own statements, this finding was so surprising for him that he devoted himself in extensive interviews to the scarce third of women who remained healthy with the aim of deciphering the "secret" of their health (which is also the title of one of his books). In the process, a deep emotional conviction of the meaningfulness of one's own life turned out to be a decisive protective factor for health among other factors. Antonovsky describes this as a feeling,

» (...) that life makes sense emotionally,, that at least some of the problems and demands posed by living are worth investing energy in, are worthy of commitment and engagement, are challenges that are "welcome" rather than burdens that one would much rather do without. This does not mean that someone high on meaningfulness is happy about the death of a loved one, the need to undergo serious operation, or being fired. But when these unhappy experiences are imposed on such a person, he or she will willingly take up the challenge, will be determined to seek meaning in it, and will do his best to overcome it with dignity. (Antonovsky, 1988, p. 18–19).

Dealing with and clarifying one's own values and goals can strengthen this sense of meaningfulness. By dealing with our personal goals we take a step back, so to speak, from the everyday stressors of the present and develop a perspective that goes beyond the current everyday life. This is especially helpful whenever we have the feeling that we are "sinking" into our daily routine due to the amount of everyday demands. The clarification and definition of one's own goals can help here to find one's own priorities and to act accordingly in the present everyday life.

Distance to the stress of everyday life

Against the backdrop of attractive goals and a positive concept of the future, stress-related evaluations of everyday demands can also change in such a way that they can be perceived more as challenges on the way to the goal. With goals in mind, one's own stress tolerance and willingness to confront unpleasant, strenuous situations increase.

Increased stress tolerance

People who experience their current everyday life as having little meaning, or those who have experienced a loss of meaning in connection with events of loss (death, divorce, illness, unemployment), can also gain a new orientation towards meaning by dealing with goals and the future. By creating meaning and identity, goals themselves represent an important resource for coping with stress.

Overcoming experiences of loss

In the following, I will give you some suggestions for your personal engagement with the question of what is really important to you (▶ Box 6.4). We find valid answers to this question not so much through strained or strictly logical reflection as through contemplative reflection, in which we feel or listen attentively within ourselves.

Box 6.4: Suggestions for Self-reflection: What Is Really Important to Me
— **The good fairy:** Imagine that a good fairy comes to you overnight. And you get the unique chance that this fairy will grant you three wishes.
  – What three wishes do you tell the magic fairy?
  – What would it look like in concrete terms if your wishes were fulfilled?

6

- **The 1 million euro question:** Imagine you had won the main prize of 1 million euros.
  - What would you do with the money?
  - Would you change your life? How?
- **Obituary:** Imagine that a few years after your death, your favourite grandson (or a good former colleague, or a friend...) writes an obituary for you.
  - What are the three most important things (qualities, accomplishments, deeds ...) about you and about your life that should be in this obituary?
- **"Youthful dreams":** Take yourself back to your youthful days.
  - What goals and ideals did you have as a teenager?
  - Which of these goals and ideals are still valid for you today?
- **Role models**
  - Which maximum of three people from your private or professional environment or from public life represent role models for you?
  - What values do these people embody for you that you would also like to realize in your own life?
- **Milestones**
  - What milestones mark your life journey so far?
  - What important decisions have you already made?
  - Which values were decisive for this?
  - What previous deeds or successes fill you with pride?

Looking Ahead: Developing a Positive Vision for the Future

» Who does not know where he wants to sail, no wind is the right one for him. (Seneca, Roman poet and philosopher, 4 B.C.–65 A.D.)

Tunnel vision in everyday life

In stress, a concentration of all physical and mental forces takes place for a confrontation with the situation that is assessed as dangerous. In the case of an acute stress situation, this is a sensible reaction. In the case of chronic stressful situations, however, as they often determine our daily and professional lives, such a reaction mode loses its meaning. We rush through our everyday life with "tunnel vision", always with the next demand in mind. We no longer notice what is happening to the left or right of us. It then happens easily that we lose direction and stray from our path without noticing it. We lose sight of our goals and can no longer recognize "favorable winds" as opportunities to realize them. We only react instead of actively shaping.

So in order not to lose orientation in stressful everyday life, it is necessary to deal from time to time with questions like: Where do I actually want to go? or: What am I doing all this for? These questions encourage us to develop a vision for the future that is as clear and positive as possible. Such a vision of the future can encompass perspectives of varying lengths, but should, as far as possible, concern a temporal zone in the future that one oneself experiences as a still manageable and meaningful section of one's own life.

Developing a vision for the future

Criteria for the definition of such an individual future space can be, for example, round birthdays, anniversaries, the end of an education, the last instalment of the mortgage loan, and so on. It should be a future perspective that on the one hand points clearly beyond the present everyday life, but on the other hand is not too broad, so that the development of a vivid idea of the future is possible. Most people choose a time frame between one and five years.

Determine personal future space

When you develop your personal vision for, think about the different areas of your life. Especially if in your present life, individual areas of life are overemphasized and others underemphasized, then your vision for the future can also be about finding a new balance of the areas of life. The distinction between the following four areas of life is useful for most people:

Observe the balance of the areas of life

Work/ performance	Tasks, projects, career, income, influence, security ...
Family/home	Partnership, children, everyday family life, parents, siblings, "nest-building" ...
Community/ contact	Friendships, belonging to a group, club member-ship, voluntary work
Person	Hobbies, sports, health, what I personally want to experience, learn, develop

The following guide (▶ Box 6.5) aims to give you some ideas for developing your personal vision of the future.

Box 6.5: View in the Future
Find a quiet place. Sit down comfortably. Inhale and exhale forcefully a few times, releasing tension from your body as you exhale.
- Imagine entering a time machine. You are embarking on a journey through time, a journey into the future, into your future. The journey takes you exactly to the time in which you have realized your next step into the future. And you

6

see there how your life looks now, when everything has gone the way you want it to.

- Look around you, at this time in your future. See what there is to discover. Look in peace. And look in all directions...
- **To your work.** What do you do for a living now? Look what's there ... What does your daily work consist of? What do you accomplish? What are you proud of? What is your professional status? What is the importance of profession and work in your life?
- **On your home** and on the people who are there. Look what is there and who is there ... Do you live in a partnership? How do you form your family relationships: with your partner, with children, with parents, and other family members? What is the importance of the family, the home community in your life?
- **To your social environment.** Where do you belong? ... What friendships or acquaintances do you maintain? How important are friends and acquaintances in your life?
- And also look **at yourself.** What about you personally? How have you developed? ... What are your personal interests? What about your hobbies? How about your self-realization? What do you do just for yourself? What new experiences have you had? What have you learned, experienced, witnessed that enriches you and fulfills you personally?
- Finally, look at your life as a whole again after your next future step.
- Memorize your pictures well. You may want to take a few more photos in your mind ...

When you want to finish the exercise, clench your hands into fists, stretch, and take a few deep breaths.

After your "view in the future", please take time to record the ideas and images that have arisen in you in the process. Write down or draw what your positive vision of your next step into the future looks like.

From the Vision to the Goal: Formulating Goals Correctly

Translating vision into goals

If you have developed a clear positive vision of your next step into the future, then you already have an important inner resource that you can fall back on in everyday life and that can give you orientation and support, especially in stressful times. However, in order for the vision not to remain a vision, but to become reality if possible, it is helpful to translate the vision into goals that you set for yourself. Goals formulate—more binding than a vision—what you intend to do in order to get closer to the vision. I sometimes see people shy away from this step because you fear that goals will only put them under further stress. However, this usually only applies to poorly formulated goals that are, for example, too vague, too unrealistic, or simply "pious wishes". Motivational psychologists have dealt intensively with the question of how goals should be formulated so that they are as motivating as possible and have a high probability of being realized. The most important criteria of a good goal formulation are:

High Personal Attractiveness

This sounds banal, but it is enormously important: goals are all the more motivating the more personally attractive they are. You can tell how attractive a goal really is for you by how much it triggers positive feelings in you, such as (pre-)joy and pleasure. This contrasts with goals that are purely driven by reason, which are emotionally neutral or even associated with negative feelings such as fear and guilt.

Anticipation has a motivating effect

Approach Goals Instead of Avoidance Goals

The goals should be formulated positively. They should include what you want to achieve. For example, "I have good contact with my children on a regular basis". Avoidance goals, on the other hand, are worded negatively and include what you want to avoid. For example, "I have fewer arguments with my children". Like a magnet, avoidance goals keep drawing your thoughts back to the negative. Well-worded approach goals, on the other hand, are associated with pleasant feelings, invigorate, and uplift.

Formulate goals positively

Action Goals Instead of Desired Goals

Action goals are goals that can be achieved through one's own actions. Action goals include the activities that one can and will undertake oneself to achieve the desired state. For example, "I will contact my children regularly". Desire goals, on the other hand, are goals whose fulfillment depends on external influences, the behaviour of others, and perhaps chance.

goals to be achieved by one's own doing

Desire goals involve positive states, but no actions of one's own to achieve them. For example, "My children keep in touch with me regularly". Action goals, on the other hand, formulate one's own possibilities, one's own readiness, and one's own will to achieve the goal.

Concrete and Verifiable

Formulate goals as concretely as possible

Instead of vague declarations of intent, the goals should be formulated as concretely as possible. So instead of "do more sports", be specific and "go swimming twice a week". Instead of "having more time for myself", you should specifically "plan half an hour a day for me to read (or listen to music, go for a walk ...)". Instead of "take more care of my friends" specifically "make a date once a week". If you formulate your goals in concrete terms, then it will also be possible to check the extent to which they have been achieved. To this end, in the formulation of your goals, you specify binding times at which you will begin certain actions or at which you want to have achieved certain interim goals. In this way you can give yourself a sense of achievement, make adjustments to your goals if necessary, and learn over time to set realistic goals (see next point).

Realistic Probability of Success

Set realistic goals

Goals can be ambitious, but they should also remain realistic. Otherwise they lead to disappointment, constant frustration, and a waste of time and energy. Here it is important to check self-critically how realistic it is to achieve the goal through one's own efforts. As a rule of thumb, goals with a probability of success of 70-80% are particularly motivating.

In a nutshell, this means:

> **Important**
> Good goals are
> — Personally attractive,
> — Put in a positive way,
> — Achievable through one's own actions,
> — Concrete, scheduled and thus verifiable,
> — Realistic.

> **My Goals by .... (Year)**
> Please formulate a maximum of three goals that will bring you closer to realizing your positive vision of the future. Think of your different areas of life and consider the criteria of good goal formulation

Important or Urgent? Set Priorities

» Along with the noble art of doing things, there is the noble art of leaving things undone. (Asian proverb)

Setting priorities is the most important rule for gaining time sovereignty and thus the possibility of getting closer to the realization of one's own goals. The distinction between importance and urgency of tasks has proven its worth. You may be familiar with the phrase: important things are rarely urgent and urgent things are rarely important. The importance of a task comes from its relevance to one's goals. Things that contribute to achieving one's goals are important. How important certain things are defined by yourself.

Important is more important than urgent!

The urgency of a task refers to the time period in which the task must be completed. Urgency is often defined by others. Urgent tasks are often important to others, not necessarily to you. Of course, important tasks can also become urgent, for example, when a certain deadline is approaching.

Being able to distinguish between the importance and urgency of a task is of great importance for setting priorities. People who are under stress and time pressure often feel that all their tasks are equally important and urgent. They are under the "tyranny of the urgent". However, a closer look usually reveals that not all urgent tasks are important at the same time.

Tyranny of the urgent

Importance and urgency influence priority setting in equal measure. If we distinguish between low and high importance or urgency, we arrive at the four-field table (Fig. 6.3). Incidentally, this is attributed to the former US president Dwight D. Eisenhower and is therefore also referred to as the Eisenhower principle.

"Eisenhower Principle"

Using this chart, you can divide all your professional and personal tasks into four priority levels.

6

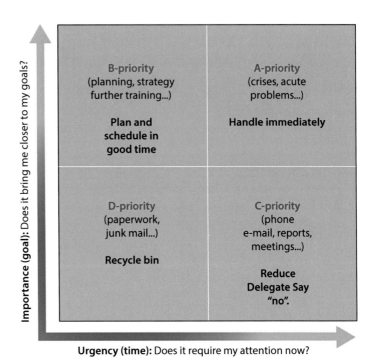

Urgency (time): Does it require my attention now?

◻ **Fig. 6.3** Setting priorities according to the "Eisenhower principle"

A-Priority

The highest priority is given to tasks in the first quadrant that are both important and urgent. These can be crises, sudden problems, or tasks with an imminent deadline. Here you need to act immediately.

B-Priority

These include the tasks of the second quadrant, the important but not or not yet urgent tasks, e.g. new projects, training measures, planning tasks. These tasks do not have to be completed immediately and are therefore often put on the back burner until they themselves become urgent again. Here it is important to regularly take the time to work on these B-tasks, because it is exactly these B-tasks that are the basis of your success in the long term and bring you closer to your goals.

C-Priority

This is about the urgent but not or less important things (third quadrant) such as some mail, e-mails, calls, meetings, interruptions, requests by others, etc. How can you protect yourself from the dictates of urgency? The key is to muster the strength and courage to set clear boundaries, to say a friendly but firm "no" or "not now" when appropriate, and to delegate tasks where possible. This is the only way to protect the time for your important B-tasks, which would otherwise be lost.

D-Priority

The lowest priority are the tasks that are neither important nor urgent (fourth quadrant). One should confidently and without much ado keep oneself free of these things. For this purpose, there is the wastepaper basket (also the electronic one!) as well as the possibility to cancel or delegate when it comes to keeping appointments or certain tasks.

If priorities are set correctly, then you actively control your daily routine. You will escape the "tyranny of the urgent" and deal with the really important things. You will be less likely to get bogged down. You won't get all the things done, but you will get the important tasks done, and therefore you will ultimately be more satisfied at the end of the day.

Dealing with what is important

Plan Time Correctly

» Most time is wasted trying to save time! (Managerial wisdom)

Clear priorities help to use time **effectively,** i.e. to spend time on the right things. The right time planning can help to do this **efficiently,** i.e. with the best possible use of your own time and energy.

The aim is not to live a life filled as much as possible, but a life fulfilled as much as possible, in which there is a balance between time for work and "free" time, between time for oneself and time for others. It is about gaining the greatest possible degree of time sovereignty and aligning the use of time as much as possible with one's own professional, family, and personal goals (cf. previous section). Time planning is not an end in itself. It is not about "saving time" in order to be able to pack your own schedule even fuller. Proper time planning can help you to use your limited time for what is really important to you (B-tasks) and to create the necessary space for regeneration.

Gain time sovereignty

There are many benefits to sensible scheduling:

Advantages of good scheduling

- Planning gives you more time and saves double work.
- Planning allows you to be "on task" and takes the pressure off your brain.
- Planning allows you to switch off after work and helps you to stay calm.
- Planning allows success control.
- Planning enables freedom and is the prerequisite for flexibility (instead of chaos).

The following **practical tips** are helpful:

Plan in Writing and with a System

Plan in writing

Depending on the personal life situation, the range here extends from the simple "to-do" list to the complex schedule book.

First Things First!

High priority tasks have priority

When you create your daily or weekly schedule, the first thing you do is schedule times for high priority tasks: the important things first.

Observe Personal Performance Curve

Observe highs and lows

There is a characteristic sequence of highs and lows in the course of each person's day. Some people experience their peak performance in the morning, others don't really get going until the afternoon, and still others have two highs, one in the morning and a second later in the afternoon with an extended low over lunchtime. What time of day do you have the most energy? When do you get the best ideas? If you know your personal daily rhythm, then you can use that knowledge to best manage your daily schedule. Schedule A- and B-tasks for times when your performance is highest, the so-called prime time. Routine tasks and low-priority tasks you schedule for times before a high, when your energy level gradually rises (called "up phases"). Use the times after a high (the so-called down phases), when your energy level drops, for rest and relaxation.

> **Observe and Reflect: Do You Know Your Daily Performance Curve?**
> What does your power curve look like on an average day? Observe your energy level on several days and assess how energetic, focused, and powerful you feel at different times of the day. When do you have your performance highs, and when do you have your lows? Plot your personal performance curve on the chart in ◘ Fig. 6.4 by assessing your energy on a scale from 0 = "no energy" to 6 = "maximum energy" for the different times of the day.

ENERGY

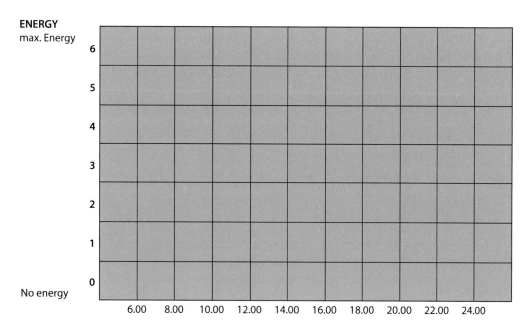

Fig. 6.4 Personal performance curve

Schedule Regular Breaks

Regular rest periods are not a useless waste of time, but important for a meaningful and effective time management, especially in times of high demands, when the pressure increases. "If you're in a hurry, go slow" is the title of a bestseller by the well-known time management expert Lothar Seiwert. The art of taking the right breaks will be discussed in more detail in ▶ Chap. 8 of this book.

Plan time for breaks

Allow for Buffer Times

Time management experts recommend keeping between 30% and 40% of your time free for unexpected and spontaneous activities or for disruptions. If you plan your time too tightly, there's a very good chance that your schedule will be upended by unpredictable things, leaving you rushed and pressed for time. "The more precise you plan, the harder chance hits you" is a common managerial wisdom. That's why it's better to plan for a little more air right from the start! That saves nerves and ultimately also time.

Keep time free for disturbances

Estimate Time Requirements Realistically

Plan time realistically

On the one hand, this means that you plan a sufficiently large period of time for individual activities, but on the other hand, it also means that you define an upper time limit for these activities. This helps to keep your own demands for perfection in check.

Follow-Up

Learning from experience

At the end of the day (or week), take a few minutes to review the extent to which you have followed your plan. This will give you a sense of achievement when you can cross off what you have done, and the opportunity to carry over what you have not done. By systematically reviewing your schedule, you can learn from your experiences and gradually adapt your schedule to the requirements and your personal daily rhythm

6

Develop Beneficial Thoughts and Attitudes: Mental Stress Competence

Contents

© Springer-Verlag GmbH Germany, part of Springer Nature 2022
G. Kaluza, *Calm and Confident Under Stress*, https://doi.org/10.1007/978-3-662-64440-9_7

> » The last of human freedoms consists in the choice of attitudes towards things.—(Viktor Frankl, Austrian psychotherapist, founder of logotherapy, 1905–1997)

Control stress aggravating thoughts

Stress arises to a considerable extent in the mind. How we assess situations and evaluate our own competencies has a great influence on whether stress occurs or not. We have discussed this in detail in the first part of this book. The second main way to cope with stress is, therefore, to be mindful of individual stress aggravating stress processing patterns and personal stress amplifiers, to reflect on them self-critically and then to develop beneficial, stress-reducing thoughts, and attitudes. This chapter deals with such possibilities of mental stress management.

Mental stress competence includes the ability to gain distance from one's own often automated stress aggravating thoughts, to question taken-for-granted evaluations of situations and one's own competencies, that is to bring movement into one's own brain and thereby allow evaluations and attitudes to emerge which have an uplifting, constructive, supportive, and motivating effect.

This is easier said than done. Personal stress amplifiers, as we have seen, are rooted in early, sometimes very early, experiences. The glasses with which we perceive situations and ourselves have (become) so much a part of ourselves that our own view often seems to us to be the only correct, indeed the only possible view. Many stress aggravating thoughts we have thought hundreds of times. They are deeply ingrained in our souls and brains and are not easily jettisoned. If you have learned to focus your attention primarily on the threatening aspects of a situation, you will eventually perceive only threatening aspects as well. The limited view confirms itself and becomes more and more entrenched. But just as we are not merely helpless victims of external circumstances, we are not merely victims of our own past experiences, our biography. We can evolve ourselves. And we can learn to get rid of the stress amplifiers, if not completely, then to gain inner distance to them and gradually soften them, and over time to develop a more constructive, beneficial mental approach to the stressors of work and everyday life.

No "naive optimism"

Here it is not about talking the word of a "naive optimism" as it is propagated by some gurus and prophets of the so-called positive thinking. These promise not only health and success but also beauty, wealth, and everlasting happiness, if one only thinks positively enough. It is suggested that everyone can think positively if he only wants to. As if you only need to flip a switch in your head and "everything will be fine". The promises of these gurus are often completely exaggerated and irredeemable. Their methods of positively reprogramming oneself with constantly repeated thoughts like "I'm good!", "I'm getting better every day!", "I can do it!" and the like are of little real use to anyone except those who sell them. Stress aggravating thought patterns and attitudes are not sustainably changed in this way, at best they are pushed back or covered up in the short term.

We cannot just take off our usual glasses, we cannot just turn off the thoughts and resolve to "stop thinking about …". That does not work and usually only leads to getting even more entangled in these thoughts. But we can distance ourselves inwardly from our thoughts, observe them with an inner distance, not let them completely dominate our feelings and actions, and recognize them for what they are, namely only thoughts and not reality. Instead of allowing ourselves to be completely dominated by the thought "I can't do that" in our feelings and actions, for example, we go at an inner distance and say to ourselves: "I am observing that I am having the thought right now: I can't do this".

So mental stress management is not about actively fighting negative, brooding, or worrying thoughts because you want them to go away, or even condemning yourself for such thoughts, but about distancing yourself inwardly and being mindful of these thoughts—and then confidently letting them pass.

Observing one's own stress thoughts with an inner distance can already reduce a lot of stress. Those who have gained such an inner distance can then go one step further to promote new, beneficial thought patterns in their brain and gradually anchor them. However, this cannot be done at the push of a button, but only step by step and requires practice—in other words, mental training!

A consistently rose-tinted view and the naïve-optimistic belief that things in life will work out well may have a positive short-term effect on how we feel, but such a view is not very helpful for dealing with stressors and strains in a way that is successful and promotes health in the long term. I learned a different understanding of optimism from the Viennese psychiatrist and psychotherapist Viktor Frankl, who gained worldwide recognition as the founder of his own psychotherapy discipline, logotherapy. According to Frankl, optimism consists in making the best (= optimum) out of a situation. Ultimately, this is exactly the goal of mental stress management. A competent mental approach to stress essentially comprises the following four aspects (◘ Fig. 7.1):

Optimism comes from optimum

- Accepting reality,
- Challenge instead of threat: Evaluate requirements constructively,

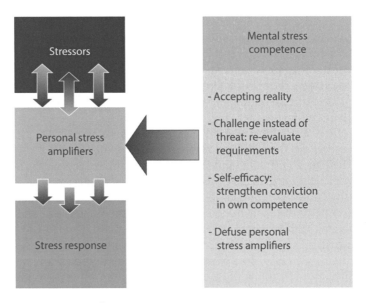

:black_small_square: **Fig. 7.1**   Mental stress competence

— Self-efficacy: strengthening the conviction in one's own competence,
— Defuse personal stress amplifiers.

Not every mental strategy that I will present to you below is useful or applicable for everyone in every situation. Again, pick and choose what is helpful for you personally.

7.1 Accepting Reality: Simple and Yet So Difficult

» What is, is, and only how I deal with it is my contribution to life.—(Lao Tzu, legendary Chinese philosopher, 6th century B.C.)

Accepting reality

Accepting reality ("That which is, that is …")—this means accepting the situation as it is—as part of my job, as part of my life. Anger, accusations, and guilt do not help any more than looking away and refusing to believe. In the first part of this book (7 ▶ Chap. 4) you have become acquainted with the stress aggravating "That can't be true!" thinking. Accepting reality interrupts this pattern of thinking.

Acceptance makes free

Accepting the situation involves two things: firstly, noticing stress signals as early as possible, and secondly, making a clear and conscious decision in favour of acceptance and thus against struggling with reality. It is precisely in this decision that our freedom lies. In the end, it is always our decision how much we let ourselves be annoyed, upset, or depressed by an external situation. And at the same time, in the decision to accept, there is also a liberation. We become freer, because we no longer spend our energy in complaining and getting angry, in fighting against and denying.

Acceptance refers both to the external stressors and to one's own physical, emotional, and mental stress reactions. Acceptance does not really change anything yet, but it prevents you from getting even more agitated and only enables you to deal constructively with the respective demands of the situation. Acceptance opens up a way out of the vicious circle that is driven by stress through stress, anger over anger, fear over fear.

Acceptance promotes stress tolerance. The well-known American psychotherapist Marsha Linehan (1996, p. 124) writes about this:

Stress tolerance

» Stress tolerance is the ability to be aware of one's surroundings without expecting them to be different, the ability to be aware of one's current emotional state without trying to change it, and the ability to observe one's thoughts and patterns of action without trying to stop or control them.

It is, therefore, a matter of an attitude of non-judgement, which, however, is not to be equated with an approval or endorsement. This is important to emphasize. Accepting reality is not the same as approving of reality. Accepting is also not the same as acquiescing or passively tolerating the situation. On the contrary, it is often only through acceptance that we regain the freedom to act constructively. Only when we face reality with a basic attitude of acceptance do we often succeed in (re)discovering and seizing our own possibilities for action.

Accepting does not mean acquiescing

What Can This Acceptance Look Like in Concrete Terms?

A few years ago, when I started giving lectures outside my familiar academic milieu in front of larger audiences, I regularly developed a very dry mouth, especially in the first few minutes of the lecture, which severely hindered my ability to speak. I was very excited before the lecture situations, which were new to me, and my body produced correspondingly large amounts of adrenaline, which resulted in the extreme dry mouth. I was aware of these connections in principle, but in the specific situations I tried to ignore and overplay them, partly because I was embarrassed to show such violent stress reactions as an expert in stress management. In the minutes leading up to the lecture, I would watch the moisture levels

Examples

7

in my mouth in anxious anticipation, with the result that the dry mouth became increasingly severe. I have since learned to embrace these strong stress reactions as part of my preparation for the task at hand. I am also no longer afraid to take a sip of water during my presentation, even in front of larger audiences, and take this as an opportunity to explain to my audience about adrenaline and physical stress reactions. Precisely because I do not simply ignore my stress reactions and do not get additionally upset or angry because of them either, but accept them as part of my reality, I can now see that the stress reactions have not completely disappeared (which would not make sense at all), but their intensity has decreased significantly.

Accepting basic attitude

A young golfer, whom I accompanied for some time as a mental coach, repeatedly complained in our meetings that he always had so much bad luck in tournaments. Especially with the short balls, which he could actually hole safely, it happened to him again and again that the ball just missed the hole due to unevenness in the ground or the like. He then gets terribly angry about his bad luck, hits the ground with his club and sometimes snaps at teammates, spectators, or his caddy. He then has one thought in particular in his head: "That can't be true!" During our conversation, it quickly became clear to him that this violent anger reaction would have a negative effect on his next tee shot and the rest of his game, and that he would no longer be able to exploit his true performance potential. When I asked him what thought could be helpful to him in such situations, he finally said with a liberating laugh after some thought: "There's that!" Such situations, he said, were actually part of the game of golf and made up part of its fascination. With this change from the "There's no such thing!" to the "There's such a thing!" thought, he had found an accepting basic attitude and had left behind the struggling with what is. Out of this accepting basic attitude, it was then also possible for him to analyse the described "bad luck situations" more precisely and to recognize that it was by no means always "bad luck", but that he also had to work on his short game.

"Shit happens"

Some time ago, I was called in for an interview by the deputy head of one of my daughters' schools. After the interview, on my way out, I saw a sign posted at eye level on the office door that led out to the school hallway that read, "Shit happens!" When I asked my interviewer about this sign, he explained that as the assistant principal, he was the school's "trouble shooter". When he left his office, he said, he always had to expect to be confronted with major or minor unforeseen difficulties and problems. When he sees the sign before he steps out into the hallway, it helps him to exhale deeply for a moment and then step out with more composure to face the challenges at hand. It helps him to accept "trouble shooting" as an important part of his task as deputy headmaster.

Observation and Reflection

Please think about concrete stressful situations from your professional or personal everyday life recently. These can be lighter and more acute situations such as being stuck in a traffic jam, having to wait at the checkout counter or on the platform, having lost something, etc., or more severe and longer-lasting stresses such as the failure of machines or employees, difficulties with pubescent children, illness, and pain in yourself or your relatives, etc.

Then please check the following questions:

- What does "accepting reality" mean in this specific stressful situation?
- To what extent does "acceptance" in this situation represent the first step towards constructive coping?

7.2 Challenge Instead of Threat: Evaluating Requirements Constructively

Beyond acceptance, mental stress competence also includes the ability to constructively evaluate demands and difficulties. This involves questioning taken-for-granted evaluations of events and developing new perspectives. Instead of one-sided perception and generalization of negative, threatening or damaging aspects, we focus our attention specifically on positive aspects of the situation in question, on the opportunities that lie within them, on the meaning that the situation can have for us, and on the positive consequences that can also result from it. In the first part of this book (▶ Sect. 4.2), you learned about stress-exacerbating thinking patterns such as "looking at the negative", "negative-consequences thinking", and "personalizing thinking". How can we reduce these stress-exacerbating thought patterns and develop stress-reducing, beneficial ways of looking at things instead? We will deal with this question in the following section.

Question evaluations, develop new perspectives

First of all, please take your time to look at the picture in ▢ Fig. 7.2. What do you recognize in this picture? Memorize this picture as well as possible. Now turn your attention once again to the picture. If you recognized an old woman in the picture before, then please try to see a young woman now. And vice versa: if you saw a young woman first, you should now see an old woman. You will find that this is not so easy. You have to make a deliberate effort to find another point of view.

Seek other points of view

7

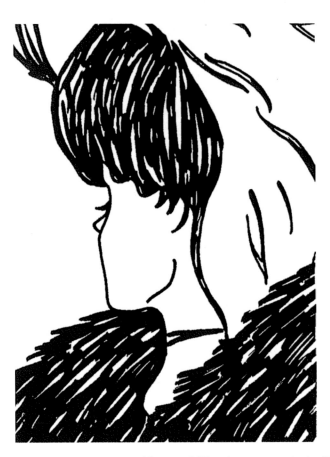

◘ **Fig. 7.2** Young woman or old woman? What do you recognize in this picture?

The first image we have gained has really taken root in our brain and is reproduced by it over and over again. If we want to recognize the other image, which is also contained in the picture, then this usually only succeeds if we literally look at it from a different angle, for example, by tilting our head or turning the picture upside down. (Here's a little help: the old woman's chin is the young woman's cleavage, the old woman's mouth becomes the young woman's collar, the old woman's nose becomes the young woman's lower jaw, and the old woman's eye becomes the young woman's ear. Try it once :-)

It is very similar with the perception and evaluation of demands. Here, too, different interpretations are often possible. And here, too, we need to make a conscious effort to overcome entrenched patterns of perception and to gain a new perspective. We often approach the demands of work and everyday life with preconceived images that have become fixed in our brains and shape our perception. They represent the glasses with which we go through our everyday life and with which we perceive and assess demands. How can we succeed in creating new perspectives in our brain so that everyday demands appear in a different light and we can perceive positive aspects and opportunities more readily?

This is not an easy task. There is no button to push to "turn on" stress-reducing, constructive perspectives in the brain. But we can question entrenched evaluations and stimulate more constructive views by asking ourselves questions. In doing so, we are, in a sense, entering into a dialogue with ourselves or with the stress-exacerbating evaluations that have become lodged in our minds. We are trying to get movement in our minds. Depending on the type of situation and the nature of our evaluation patterns, different questions can be helpful. In the following, I will show the questioning strategies that have proven particularly effective in practice for different people.

Enter into a dialogue with yourself

View at the Positive

The point here is to focus our attention on the opportunities and meaning that the situation in question can also have for us and our lives, instead of perceiving the threatening or harmful aspects of the situation in a one-sided way. This does not mean that we should gloss over a stressful situation or look at everything through rose-tinted glasses. Rather, it means that in spite of all the negativity, one should always look at the things in one's own life that are pleasing, successful, or beautiful. Demands can always be a challenge for learning and opportunities for personal development. In order to do this, it may be necessary to widen the narrow tunnel vision that one often has during stress and to look beyond the current situation. This can then lead to stress and anger fading away and feelings of satisfaction, pride, and gratitude emerging. If we also widen our gaze to see the positive, then this can also remind us of those situations that we may have initially judged to be unambiguously and exclusively negative, but which in hindsight may well have had positive aspects or personal meaning. There is the proverbial "good luck in bad luck", the "good in the bad". And this realization leads us to evaluate and judge less, and to accept things as they are. It is also beneficial if you question and put into perspective the significance of the negative aspects for yourself and focus your attention on what is really important to you, that is to see what is essential.

With the following questions you can stimulate such a "View at the positive":

Check situation for chances or sense

- What is good about this situation?
- What is this—also—good for?
- Where are the opportunities?

— What can I learn in this situation?
— What is my role in this situation?
— What sense do I make of this situation?
— How important is this really to me? What is more important than this thing?
— What beautiful things have I experienced? What good things have been or will be bestowed upon me? What am I grateful for?

If you deal with such and similar questions, this can lead to the fact that in you the thought "I must ..." is replaced by the thought "I want ...". This means that you can better recognize and accept the challenges, the opportunities, and the tasks that the respective situations hold in store for you, and that you are ready to actively face these challenges.

Reality Testing and Concretization

Reality check

Sometimes we tend to give situations or other people's behaviour a personal meaning that, on reflection, they do not really have. We then get involved in something that may no longer have much to do with the original situation (see "Personalising" in ▶ Sect. 4.2). The way to reduce stress is to maintain more inner distance, to take a step back and look at the situation from a different perspective, for example, from the perspective of a neutral observer. Even if you tend to generalize negative events or experiences hastily, it can be helpful for you to bring your head back down to earth, to carry out a mental reality check and to remind yourself of the concrete initial situation that triggered the stress. The following questions serve to check the reality content of your own perception of the situation:
— What exactly happened?
— Is it always like this? Are there exceptions?
— Is it really so? What evidence/facts support my view?
— What other ways are there to explain the situation?
— How do the other people involved feel about it? How do they feel?
— How do other (neutral, independent, experienced) people see it?
— What would the events look like in a documentary film?

If you manage to occupy your mind with such questions, this can help you to gain a more realistic assessment of the situation, to see things more clearly again. You will probably no longer see the situation itself as so threatening and as easier to handle.

Relativizing and Distancing

If you easily lose your sense of proportion, if you tend to make a mountain out of a molehill, then it is helpful for you to put things back into perspective, to put them into perspective (not to minimize them). The following questions can be helpful:

Putting the situation into perspective

- How will I feel about it later, in a month or a year?
- What does someone less burdened by the situation than me think?
- How important is this thing really to me? What is more important than this thing?
- What does the situation look like from a higher vantage point?

If you manage to occupy your mind with such questions, this will probably lead to you being able to see more clearly again what is essential, what is really important to you. The questions can also help you to gain more inner distance especially if you tend to take things too personally (▶ Chap. 4, ▶ Sect. 4.2).

Positive Consequences Thinking

In the first part of this book (▶ Sect. 4.2), you learned about negative consequence thinking as a stress-exacerbating thought pattern. Instead of thinking about the negative consequences of failing to meet a challenge, we can focus our attention on the possible positive consequences of meeting it successfully. We then envision in great detail what it will be like when we have mastered the situation at hand. This is not to superficially tell ourselves that "everything will be fine". It is rather a matter of directing our gaze to possible successes and opportunities that the requirement also holds in store for us and imagining as vividly as possible what it will be like when we have mastered the situation. This does not mean completely ignoring the risks and dangers, but also perceiving the opportunities. Instead of fear of failure, this creates hope for success, strength, and motivation. Here, too, it is beneficial to question and put into perspective the actual significance of the expected negative consequences for oneself and to reflect on the essentials. Sometimes it can also be helpful if you mentally play through the feared catastrophic consequences to the very end. This then often leads to decatastrophizing, that is the realization that one will ultimately survive despite all the dire consequences.

Think of positive consequences

This also requires practice and targeted stimulation of the brain, which all too easily tends to get lost in preoccupation with feared negative consequences. Dealing with the following questions can help:

— What will it be like when I have successfully completed the requirement?
— How will that make me feel?
— How will others I care about react to my success?
— How will this positively affect my life situation?
— Also de-catastrophize:
— What would happen at worst? How bad would that really be? How likely is that?

Let "pictures of success" arise in your mind that are as vivid as possible. This will help you to experience the respective requirements less as a threat and instead to feel strength, motivation, and possibly even joy within yourself.

Practice constructive thinking

If you are trying to get things moving in your head with these and similar questions in order to overcome one-sided and entrenched patterns of perception and evaluation and to gain new constructive perspectives, then beware of giving up too quickly. Stay persistent. Your brain must first become accustomed to these new questions; the corresponding neural circuits must first be created and developed through frequent use until they are so strong that they can replace the old patterns formed through years of use (see also the explanations on neural plasticity in ▶ Sect. 2.6).

> **Train Supportive Thinking**
> If you have the impression that stress aggravating thinking also plays a role in your personal stress experience, then you should systematically train your brain in beneficial thinking. To do this, choose one or two questions from the possibilities listed above and ask yourself these questions regularly, preferably at a specific time each day. For example, if you have a one-sided tendency to "look at the negative", ask yourself the question, "What was good today?" every evening. If "negative-consequence thinking" is strong in your mind, then you can present yourself with the question, "What will go well today?" every morning, for example. In this way, you can train your brain in beneficial, stress-reducing thinking. And as with any training, the same is true here: only patient, regular, repeated practice over a long period of time will lead to success.

7.3 Self-efficacy: The Conviction of One's Own Competence

Stress always arises when we do not trust ourselves to successfully cope with a requirement. In addition to the assessment of the respective demands, it is, therefore, always also a question of an assessment of our own competencies. It is possible that we actually lack the necessary competencies to be able to successfully master a given challenge. In this case, we are rightly under stress, so to speak.

Importance of own competences

Often, however, we lack an objective benchmark or we simply do not trust ourselves to do it. We underestimate our abilities; we lack confidence in our own competence. In the first part of this book you got to know "deficit thinking" (► Sect. 4.2) as a pattern of stress aggravating thinking. It consists of focusing attention too one-sidedly on one's own weaknesses, mistakes, and failures. The beneficial, stress-reducing alternative here is to think in terms of **strengths**, which leads to self-acceptance. This is not about superficially telling yourself "You can do it!". Rather, strengths thinking means becoming aware of one's strengths, competencies and successes and remembering past difficult situations that one has already mastered. However, not only memories of situations in which things went well for us, but also experiences with past situations that were associated with defeats and failures, but which we somehow overcame in the end, can be helpful here. They also strengthen one's own conviction of self-efficacy, the deep trust in one's own strength to be able to get through even difficult situations. Incidentally, thinking in terms of strengths does not mean, as is sometimes misunderstood, that one suppresses or denies one's own weaknesses as far as possible, but that one perceives and accepts oneself with one's weaknesses and strengths ("I am good the way I am".).

Self-efficacy: "I can do it"

Health psychologists also speak of **self-efficacy** in this context. This refers to a deep, inner conviction that one can cope with difficult situations on one's own, especially when one cannot be one hundred percent sure that one really can due to previous experiences. It is, therefore, an optimistic confidence in one's own abilities and strengths, it is the "I can do it" conviction. Numerous scientific studies have repeatedly shown that a high self-efficacy belief makes it easier to cope with everyday stress.

How Can We Gain Such an Optimistic Self-efficacy Belief?

Self-efficacy comes from experience

Many of you will share the experience that it is of little use if we try to convince ourselves of the "I can do it" conviction like a prayer mill. Even good coaxing from others ("You can do it ...") usually only has a short-term effect. Sustainable self-efficacy is ultimately based on experience. Experiences with difficult situations in our lives, which we—in whatever way— have mastered. Most people can look back on such experiences, however the memories of them are often buried and overlaid by memories of experiences of failure that most of us have also had. This is where it comes down to consciously bringing to mind the memories of those situations where we succeeded at something that we were not initially convinced we could succeed at. These experiences are the food for self-efficacy beliefs. We need to keep them awake and alive in us (▶ Box 7.1).

> **Box 7.1: Remembering and Reflecting**
> To stimulate "strengths thinking", take a moment to consider the following questions:
> - What difficult situations in my life have I already mastered or gotten through? How did I manage to do that?
> - What strengths and virtues have I demonstrated in the process?
> - What am I proud of?
> - What gives me courage and security today? What can I rely on?
> - How would a good friend (or colleague, father, mother, someone who "has my back") describe my strengths?

Gaining confidence in one's own competence

Just like trust in other people, trust in one's own competence grows step by step with experience. However, such growth does not happen by itself. In order for trust between people to grow, it requires the courage of each individual to take a step towards the other and thus accept the risk of disappointment or rejection. Without such courage to take calculated risks, trusting relationships between people cannot develop. It is quite similar with the growth of trust in one's own competence. Here, too, we need the courage to take a new step, to face a new challenging situation and to accept the risk of failure. We need to overcome the fear of failure. When we muster this courage, we enable ourselves to have the very experiences that confidence in our own competence needs in order to grow.

Namely, the experience of having successfully applied one's own competencies in a new, uncertain situation.

Of course, experiences of failure are also possible, but these can also be used to strengthen self-efficacy if we analyse them carefully. Did I take on too much? What about my approach contributed to the failure? What was the reason I did not achieve my goal? If we answer these questions honestly, we can learn from a failure experience. And we learn to process failure better. After all, it is not the failure itself that undermines our confidence in ourselves, but the fear of failure and its consequences. In this respect, the experience of failure and especially the experience of having "survived" a failure, perhaps even having grown from it, can contribute to a strengthening of the self-efficacy conviction.

"Nothing ventured, nothing gained". This saying, therefore, also applies when it comes to strengthening our own self-efficacy convictions. However, this does not mean that we should expose ourselves to incalculable risks without appropriate preparation. In order to increase the probability of a successful experience, it is important to have good mental preparation. Here we can make use of the human brain's ability to anticipate situations. Instead of thinking about the possible negative outcomes of a situation, as is often the case, we use our ability to anticipate in order to imagine as vividly and in as much detail as possible how we will act successfully in the challenging situation in question. We develop within ourselves a script for our "success story". In mental training for athletes, such a procedure has been practiced for a long time, in which athletes repeatedly mentally imagine the correct movement sequences in preparation for a competition or even during a competition. Such an "inner film" of one's own action steps, which is as vivid as possible, is extremely helpful when it comes to actual action in a concrete situation (▶ Box 7.2).

Dealing with failure constructively

Mental training

> **Box 7.2: Imagination Exercise: "Successful Coping"**
> Think of an upcoming challenging situation (e.g. a difficult client meeting, a public appearance, a critique meeting with a co-worker, an exam, a contentious family dispute, etc.). Make as detailed a plan as possible for how you will proceed, what you will do or say, and how. Then close your eyes and picture in your mind's eye all the details of how you will successfully meet the challenge. Memorize this inner image and the good feelings associated with it as deeply as possible.
>
> Repeat this idea until you can reliably recall the image and feeling of successful mastery.

7.4   Defusing Personal Stress Amplifiers: The Development Square

Motives behind the stress amplifiers

In the first part of this book, you learned about five common personal stress amplifiers and that they ultimately consist of an exaggeration of normal human needs or desires (▶ Sect. 4.3). For example, the "Be perfect!" amplifier is based on the achievement motive, the "Be popular!" amplifier is based on the attachment motive, the "Be independent!" amplifier is based on the autonomy motive, the "Stay in control" amplifier is based on the control motive, and the "Hang in there" amplifier is based on the protection motive. When these general human motives are made absolute, when their fulfillment is exaggerated into an absolute must, then this makes us stress-prone to all those situations in which it is questionable whether the respective motive can be fulfilled. Even more, we will then interpret a multitude of everyday situations as a threat to this motive.

How can personal stress amplifiers be defused? As always when it comes to personal development, self-awareness is the first step. It is important to recognize one's own individual stress amplifier profile and to admit the individual susceptibilities to stress caused by this (see ◘ Fig. 4.3 in ▶ Chap. 4).

Too much of a good thing

"In my job, absolute accuracy is important, so you have to be a bit of a perfectionist", "I just feel good when everything is harmonious and everyone likes me", "It's good to have everything under control yourself instead of relying on others", "I just like being there for others, and I want to keep it that way", something like that are often the first reactions of seminar participants when the topic of personal stress intensifiers and ways to change them comes up. These statements quite rightly express that the attitudes and behaviours associated with stress amplifiers are not only bad, that they also have much good in them. Therefore, when we address the question of how to defuse personal stress amplifiers, this cannot be a matter of simply throwing the stress amplifiers overboard. That would hardly be possible, nor would it make sense. Rather, it is important to preserve the positive aspects of the respective attitudes and behaviours and at the same time to reduce the negative, that is the stress-producing aspects.

Development square

In order to see things more clearly here, we can make use of a mental tool presented by the Hamburg psychology professor Friedemann Schulz von Thun: the so-called development square. It assumes that the value of behaviours, virtues, or attitudes is always relative. Every strength can become a weakness, and that is precisely when one does too much of a

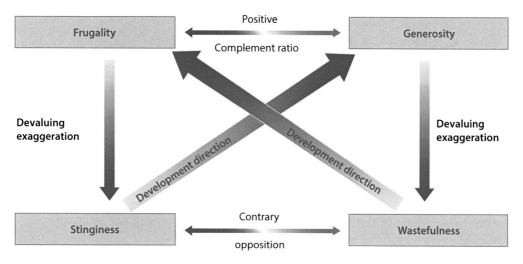

☐ Fig. 7.3 Development square using the example of "thriftiness". (Adapted from Schulz von Thun 1989)

good thing. Frugality then becomes stinginess, and courage becomes overconfidence. In order to avoid the danger of such a devaluing exaggeration, it is necessary that the respective attitudes and behaviours are in a good balance with a complementary behaviour or attitude, that there is an opposite pole in each case. In the case of frugality, for example, the opposite pole would be generosity; in the case of courage, it would be prudence. This opposite pole, too, bears the danger of a devaluing exaggeration. Generosity then becomes wastefulness and prudence slips into cowardice. We can represent these considerations in the form of a square, as illustrated in ☐ Fig. 7.3 using the example of thrift. The two complementary positive qualities (in the example, thrift and generosity) are at the top. They are in a positive relationship of tension and together form a unit. The corresponding devaluing exaggerations (stinginess and wastefulness) form the two lower corners of the square. They form a contrary opposition. They occur when the value in the opposite upper corner of the square is missing.

Now we can also see the direction in which personal development should take place. For a person who tends to exaggerate frugality, it is a matter of learning to be generous once in a while without falling into the other extreme, wastefulness. Conversely, someone who tends to exaggerate generosity should learn frugality without becoming stingy. This is the basic idea of the development square. It helps us to see directions of development, overcoming simple black-and-white thinking, and keeps us from falling from one extreme to the other.

Identify direction for personal development

We can now apply the development square to the five personal stress amplifiers. To do this, we ask ourselves the following questions in each case:

1. What is good about the stress amplifier? What positive qualities and behaviours are associated with the particular stress amplifier?
2. What is the devaluing exaggeration, the "too much of a good thing" in this stress amplifier?
3. What is the positive antithesis of the positive traits and behaviours described in 1?
4. What is the devaluing exaggeration in this antithesis?
5. In which direction should personal development go?

Development squares for stress amplifiers

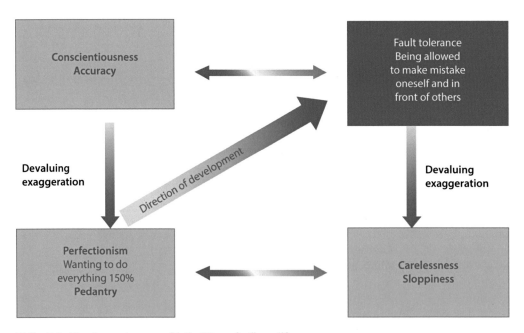 Figures 7.4, 7.5, 7.6, 7.7, and 7.8 show the development squares for the five stress amplifiers. The blue arrows indicate the direction of development for someone with a strong expression of the respective stress intensifier. If we know the direction in which we want to develop, then we can also plan the first concrete steps that lead in this direction and enable us to have new experiences. Because ultimately it is such new experiences that lead to a gradual change in overarching attitudes, to a defusing of personal stress amplifiers.

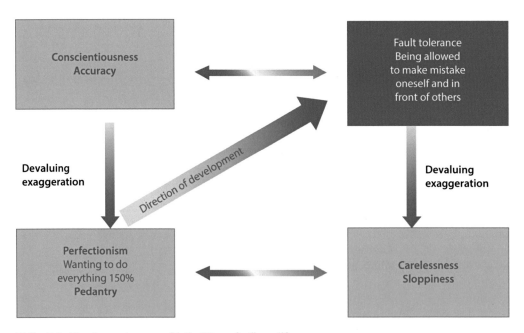

□ **Fig. 7.4** Development square with the "Be perfect" amplifier

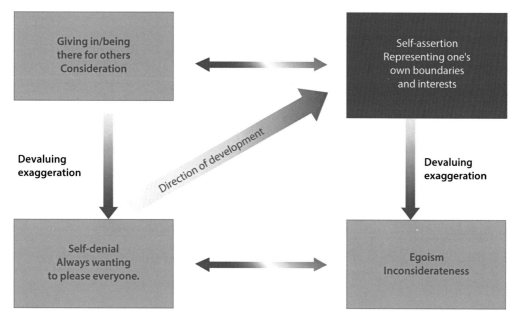

Fig. 7.5 Development square with the "Be popular" amplifier

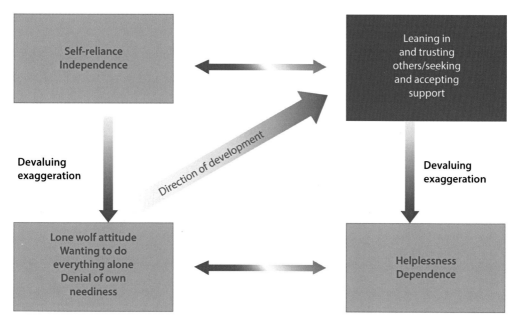

Fig. 7.6 Development square with the "Be independent" amplifier

7

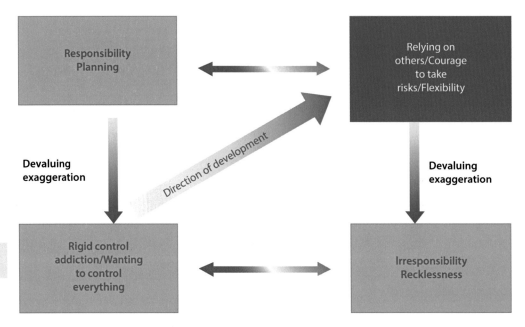

◨ **Fig. 7.7**   Development square in the "Keep control" amplifier

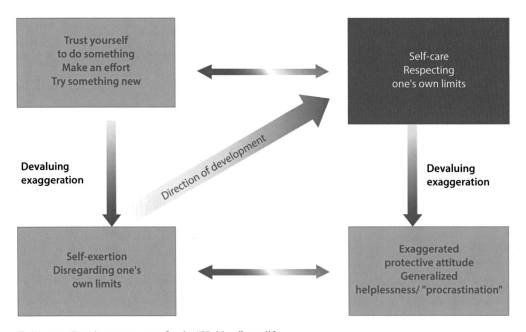

◨ **Fig. 7.8**   Development square for the "Hold on" amplifier

Development Direction of the "Be Perfect" Amplifier

For someone with a strong expression of the "Be perfect!" amplifier, it is therefore important to learn fault tolerance to allow oneself to make mistakes, inadequacies, and inaccuracies in front of oneself and in front of others, or at least to tolerate them without falling into the other extreme, namely careless-ness and sloppiness (◻ Fig. 7.4). In essence, it is a matter of allowing oneself and tolerating the fact that one also delivers a work result of which one knows that one could do even better. The first step in this direction can be, for example, setting your-self a time limit for less important tasks and being satisfied with a result that does not meet all your own demands. This can pro-vide the experience that "good" (and just not perfect) is often good enough. Being open in front of others about one's own minor mistakes or inaccuracies can also be an important step, which can convey the healing experience that others do not reject one because of this, but on the contrary may value one as a human being precisely because of this. Thoughts that can helpfully support such a path of development are, for example:

Develop fault tolerance

- I am allowed to make mistakes too.
- I learn from my mistakes.
- I am okay in spite of flaws.
- Even good/usable/80% is often good enough.
- Less is sometimes more.
- As good as possible, as good as necessary.
- Every now and then I let 5 be straight.
- I do my best and take care of myself.
- I distinguish between important and unimportant.

Development Direction of the "Be Popular" Amplifier

The "Be popular!" reinforcer is about practicing self-assertion and learning to represent one's own boundaries and interests without falling into the opposite extreme of ruthless egoism (◻ Fig. 7.5). In essence, this is about allowing oneself to dis-appoint other people once in a while and being able to endure the fact that others are not satisfied with one in all respects. The first concrete steps on this path can consist, for example,

Exercise assertiveness

of saying "no" in easier situations and to people who do not mean that much to you, or delegating tasks. The experience of getting relief in this way, without significantly straining one's relationship with others, can then lead to a gradual softening of the "Be popular!" amplifier. Thoughts that can be helpful in this process include:

- I get to say no.
- I am mindful of my boundaries/needs.
- I take care of myself too.
- I am good to myself.
- I am allowed to disappoint others.
- I am allowed to be edgy.
- I cannot/would not/have to please everyone.
- Not everyone else has to like me.
- Criticism is part of it.
- I am allowed to criticize/say my opinion.
- I am allowed to be criticized.

Development Direction of the "Be Independent" Amplifier

Accept support

Personal development lies in learning to lean on others at times and to accept support without giving up one's independence and putting oneself in a helpless-dependent position (◘ Fig. 7.6). In essence, this is about allowing oneself and being able to endure being dependent on others at times and relying on others. In concrete terms, this can mean, for example, showing someone else that you need help with a particular task and openly asking for it. This allows for the relieving experience that support from others is possible without having to "make oneself small" in the process. Thoughts that can helpfully accompany such a development process are, for example:

- I am allowed to show weakness.
- Weakness is human.
- I may ask for help/support.
- There is help/support for me.
- I give others a chance to support me.
- I am allowed to let myself go.
- I may/can delegate.
- I may/can rely on/trust others.
- I do not have to do everything myself/alone.
- I am allowed to show my feelings.
- I get to lean.

Development Direction of the "Keep Control" Amplifier

For people with a strong sense of control, it is a matter of developing the courage to take—calculated—risks and learning to engage in new, unfamiliar, unpredictable situations without becoming reckless (◘ Fig. 7.7). At its core, this is about tolerating uncertainty and allowing oneself to take risks. Not planning all the details of an upcoming event in advance for once, or controlling others less and trusting them more instead, can represent steps in this direction. This allows for experiences that gradually soften the overly caution and excessive control seeking. Supporting thoughts in this can be:

- I get to let go.
- I am allowed to take a risk.
- I dare.
- I can/may decide for this situation.
- It is good to have courage.
- I can correct decisions.
- I can/may be spontaneous.
- I can/do trust my gut.
- Risk/uncertainty is part of it.
- I can/do rely on others.
- I have faith.
- Disruptions are part of the job/plan.
- I remain calm, even though I do not know what is coming.
- No risk, no fun!

Develop the courage to take risks

Development Direction of the "Hang in There!" Amplifier

This is about self-care and paying more attention to one's own limits, without slipping into the other extreme of an exaggerated protective attitude (◘ Fig. 7.8). In essence, it is a matter of being able to allow oneself, or at least endure, to avoid an unpleasant task, to give up goals that prove to be too ambitious, to perceive and accept one's own limits, and to rest. Important steps in this direction could be, for example, to allow oneself breaks, even if one is not yet on the verge of exhaustion.

Helpful thoughts along the way might include:
- I will take care of myself.
- I will take care of myself.
- I get to rest/relax.

Respect your own limits

- I am allowed to take the easy way out.
- I get to let go.
- I am allowed to give up.
- I have boundaries, and that is good.

3 steps to personal development

To summarize, defusing personal stress amplifiers depends on three things: firstly, there is reflection and self-awareness of personal stress amplifiers and the attitudes and behaviours associated with them. Secondly, it is a matter of positively determining the direction of personal development. Here, the development square can serve us well. Thirdly, and finally, we need to take concrete small steps in our everyday lives that lead in the direction of development we have identified and enable us to have new experiences.

Stimulation for Self-reflection
- What personal attitudes and behaviours contribute to my everyday stress experience?
- What is good about these attitudes and behaviours?
- What is the devaluing exaggeration ("too much of a good thing")?
- In which direction would I like to develop personally?
- What concrete steps can I take towards this in my everyday life?

Creating Balance: Regenerative Stress Competence

Contents

© Springer-Verlag GmbH Germany, part of Springer Nature 2022
G. Kaluza, *Calm and Confident Under Stress*, https://doi.org/10.1007/978-3-662-64440-9_8

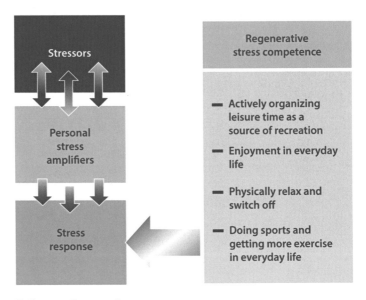

◘ Fig. 8.1   Regenerative stress competence

8

Alleviate the effects of stress, recharge your batteries

This third pillar of stress management focuses on the regulation and control of physical and mental stress reactions. It is about how we can release physical tension, dampen inner restlessness and nervousness, and provide balance in order to avoid or alleviate negative stress consequences in the long term, as well as strategies that serve to maintain our own resistance to stress and build up new energies.

Specifically, in this chapter we will look at the following four components of regenerative stress competence (◘ Fig. 8.1):

- Active recreation,
- Enjoy in everyday life,
- Relax and switch off mentally,
- Exercise and bring more movement into everyday life.

8.1 Actively Shaping Recreation

» The art of resting is part of the art of working—(John Steinbeck, American writer and Nobel Prize winner, 1902–1968)

Vicious circle: withdrawal increases feelings of stress

Under stress, many people not only tend to withdraw socially, but also to let interests wither, to give up hobbies, sports, and other leisure activities. As long as it is only a short-term, time-limited phase of stress, this can be an appropriate and promising strategy in terms of concentrating one's strengths. In the case of prolonged stress, however, such a self-restriction leads to a fatal vicious circle: stress and physical as well as psychological stress symptoms take up an ever larger part of life. The subjective feeling of stress continues to increase. Positive experiences become rarer and rarer, whereas depressive moods and feelings of anxiety increase. In the long run, the lack of opportunities for recovery and compensation leads to a further decrease in resistance to stress.

Other people fill their free time with a variety of activities, but actually do not experience any real recreation. They are stuck in the "leisure trap". They transfer the norms and criteria of the working world to their leisure time as well. Performance thinking, perfectionism, ambition, prestige, and the need to consume also determine leisure time behaviour. Hectic activity, impatience, and the fear of missing out leave no room for inner peace and leisure. Leisure time is therefore not a regenerative counter-world to working life, but rather a doubling of it. A study conducted by the Cologne Sports University in 2003, under the direction of psychology professor Henning Allmer, revealed that three out of four of the approximately 5,000 employed Germans surveyed were unable to relax and enjoy their leisure time. The balance between work and leisure, the so-called work-life balance is permanently disturbed. Leisure time also means taking time out, doing nothing for once with a clear conscience. Idleness is not, as the saying goes, the beginning of all vices. Idleness is rather the prerequisite for not wasting time, but using it for self-reflection.

"Leisure trap"

There is often a lack of awareness that daily rest is necessary to maintain one's own performance and health. In sports, it has long been accepted that top performance is based on systematic recovery training. With regard to performance in the professional and family sphere, we are still a long way from this attitude. Recovery can and should be actively managed. In the following, I would like to give you a few pointers on what is important here.

Daily rest is necessary

■ **Recover: From What?**

Perhaps you too share these experiences: After a "restful" weekend or a short vacation, you still feel stressed and drained. Despite 8 h of sleep, you are still not rested. If the hoped-for rest fails to materialize, it is often due to a misconception of rest. Many people believe that passive rest alone will bring about the desired and necessary recovery. Modern recovery research, however, shows that we do not have to wait passively for recovery alone, but that we can and must actively shape the recovery process ourselves in order to achieve the desired recovery effect.

Actively shape recreation

To do this, we need to develop a sense for signals of the need for recovery and we need to know what we actually want to recover from and for what purpose. Not all recovery is the same. Which form of recovery is the right one depends on which form of strain we have experienced before.

> ❯ Please think about this: How do you feel after a hard day's work or a long week's work?

■ **Do You Especially Feel Inwardly Restless, Exhilarated, Nervous and Overstimulated?**

Seek rest

Then your recovery is primarily about finding inner rest. Relaxing activities that reduce physical and mental activation are the optimal way to recover. Examples of this are systematic relaxation exercises, stays and walks in nature, in places of silence, in order to contain the sensory overload. Sporting endurance activities, practiced with a steady rhythm over a long period of time, can also contribute to calming down, provided they are practiced without false ambition and the will to achieve. Enjoyable social gatherings with others also contribute to relaxation, provided they do not involve new stressful demands, for example, as a host.

■ **Do You Mainly Feel Bad-Tempered, Frustrated, and Simply Fed Up?**

Balancing head and hand

Then you are probably too one-sidedly stressed in your everyday life. You should find activities for your leisure time that are suitable to stimulate your idle interests and abilities, and to compensate for one-sided strains. If you do "mental work" all day, you need physical activity to compensate. On the other hand, those who are physically challenged in their jobs should choose an activity in their free time that stimulates the mind. If, for example, you are a manager or work in a helping profession where you have to hold many conversations and can rarely look back on "tangible" results in the evening, a sensible way to compensate for this can be to create something with your hands, to become creatively active.

■ **Do You Feel Mainly Unfulfilled, Bored, or Underchallenged?**

Seek challenges

You feel less and less positive challenges in your professional and private everyday life? In your life, there is a lack of pleasurable states of tension? Then it is advisable to do something meaningful in your free time, to look for new personal challenges and to open up new fields of experience. For example, by starting to learn something new (a sport, a musical instrument, a language). Volunteering for an idea or a project that is important to you personally is also a way to overcome the "inner emptiness".

- **Do You Especially Feel Exhausted, Drained, Just Plain Exhausted?**

Then leisure time is all about resting and recharging your batteries. Allow yourself some time out in which you pamper yourself, for example, by taking a full bath, a sunbath, a sauna bath. As the Austrian actor Paul Hörbiger (1894–1981) once aptly put it, relaxation does not necessarily consist in doing nothing, but in doing what we do not normally do. If, however, what we do not do otherwise is precisely idleness, if we function in a mode of continuous activity without a break, then we find relaxation above all in idleness, in letting ourselves drift along without intention or plan, in idleness. Allow yourself to simply "do nothing" for once, to doze and let body and soul dangle. Make sure you get enough restful sleep. And treat yourself to delicious and healthy food!

Compensation: doing nothing!

- **The Art of the Pause**

It belongs to a musical composition like the notes and it is like the movement of an important element of every dance choreography. It is indispensable for any reasonably structured sports training. It is an integral part of the timetable in our schools and the subject of collective agreements: the **break**.

We need breaks to relax mind and body, to process and gain distance, to regenerate after a phase of tension, commitment, and engagement, and to find ourselves again. Regular breaks are a prerequisite for a healthy rhythm in the alternation between tension and relaxation, which ultimately constitutes vitality (see also ► Sect. 8.3). The greater the load and the greater the stress, the more intensive and deeper the relaxing breaks must be. This refers to the annual rhythm with the longer holiday breaks (Section "Relaxation and holidays" in this chapter), to the weekly rhythm with the after-work and weekend breaks (► Sect. 8.2 in this chapter) and to the daily rhythm with several shorter breaks, which will be discussed below.

We need breaks

Many people today live their professional and personal everyday lives in a non-stop mode of continuous activity. Driven by ever new external demands and internal stress amplifiers, many of us are, in a sense, constantly "online". Since no one is there to ring the bell for us, we have to set it ourselves: the break.

How can this succeed? First of all, it is important that we do not ignore the signals of the need for recovery, but that we instead develop fine antennae for the first signs of a decline in performance and concentration and then take these signs seriously. The recovery effect of short breaks is particularly high if

Take a break in good time

you allow yourself the breaks before performance and concentration noticeably decline. As a rule of thumb, you can stick to an approximate 90-min rhythm. After such a period of concentrated work, body and mind need a time out of 10–20 min.

Take the right break

Move a little and stretch your muscles. Drink and maybe have a snack. Get some fresh air. Perhaps do a short relaxation exercise (▶ Sect. 8.3 of this chapter) or do simple manual things to relax your mind and body. But avoid "abusing" your break by quickly doing something else "in between". For mind workers, it is important to let your brain rest too. Avoid cluttering the brain with "info junk" from the radio, TV, or magazines lying around during breaks. Instead, make sure that the brain can relax with positive, pleasant impressions (music, pictures, nature).

Gaining time through breaks

It is about stopping the inner urge to "work through" without a break. The conviction that you always have to complete an activity before you can take a break, or the worry that interrupting an activity will cause you to lose time, often stand in the way of this. Make yourself clear: regular rest periods are not a useless waste of time, but are important for maintaining your own performance, especially in times of high demands. If you act according to this insight, you will quickly notice that you do not lose anything by taking breaks, but gain time through higher efficiency.

Unfortunately, in many companies there is still a corporate culture in which those employees who are prepared to "work through the night", work a lot of overtime—mostly grey—and carry over the holiday days to which they are entitled unused into the next year, are still held in particularly high esteem by their superiors. The—open or secret—rewarding of such work behaviour not only endangers the health and performance of the individual employee, but also causes productivity losses and costs for the company in the long term due to sickness-related absences. The familiar phrase "healthy employees cost money, sick ones cost a fortune" applies here. A rethink on the part of HR managers and supervisors in terms of sustainable personnel care is urgently required here, not least in view of ageing workforces.

■ **Restful Sleep**

Sleep means regeneration

We sleep because we get tired. Everyone knows that. However, the actual reason why we get tired in the first place is surprisingly not yet known even by modern sleep research. Many researchers assume that fatigue occurs when certain metabolic products that accumulate in our body during the day need to be broken down. One thing is certain: sleep is probably the most important and efficient biological regeneration program we have. Sleeping serves the recovery of the organs.

After sleep, many bodily functions work better than after a longer period of wakefulness. However, the sleep program can also be easily impaired by strong or persistent stress reactions. Difficulty falling asleep or sleeping through the night is a common and serious warning sign of long-term stress. Sleep is essential for life. Rats die in animal experiments when they experience complete sleep deprivation over an extended period of 1–2 weeks. However, even severe sleep disturbances may not be so severe as to put the sufferer's life in danger.

Sleep disorders due to permanent stress

■ How Much Sleep Do I Need?

There is no universal "normal" measure of sleep. The average amount of sleep for adults is 7–8 h. However, some people feel well rested after only 5 h of sleep, while others need over 10 h to feel fresh and rested during the day. Scientists assume that the optimal amount of sleep required varies biologically from person to person and is largely determined by genetic makeup. For example, it has been possible to breed breeds of mice that sleep considerably more or less than the average mouse. However, current living conditions also influence the need for sleep. We need less sleep at times when we are highly motivated, when we frequently do sport and when everything is going well.

Just as important as the duration is the quality of sleep. In the case of people who complain about too little sleep, an examination in the sleep laboratory often reveals that these people actually sleep long enough—contrary to their own subjective impression—but that the depth of sleep leaves something to be desired. With sufficiently long and good sleep, we feel rested and pleasantly relaxed in the morning and at the same time energetic and in a good mood. Good and sufficiently long sleep increases our resilience and boosts our performance.

■ Sleep Hygiene: What Can I Do Myself for Healthy, Restful Sleep?

The term sleep hygiene refers to lifestyle habits and behaviours that promote healthy sleep. Below are the main rules recommended by sleep doctors.

Sleep hygiene rules

■ Stick to Regular Bedtimes and Wake-Up Times

If possible, go to bed at the same time every day (even on weekends) and—even more importantly—always get up at the same time so that your "inner clock" does not get out of rhythm. So heed grandmother's advice: "Always go to bed at the same time and get up at the same time, saves many a morning horror". On the other hand, the old principle of "early to bed and early to rise" only applies to morning types, but not to evening

Set "Inner Clock"

types. The key is regularity. Once you have stayed up late, there is only one thing to do to maintain your internal sleep-wake rhythm: get up at the same time. Merely sleeping longer on a single day, such as Sunday, usually does not disrupt your rhythm too much. However, there are people who react very sensitively to such a one-off deviation in rhythm, for example, with a migraine attack.

■ **Be Physically Active**

Work out

Get your circulation going regularly in the morning or early afternoon, but avoid strenuous physical activity just before bedtime. Regularly practiced sport promotes sleep, while on the other hand, lack of exercise and too little physical exertion can lead to sleep problems. However, the positive effect of exercise depends on general personal fitness and the time of day at which it is practiced. People who have good physical fitness should not exercise 6 h before bedtime. While exercise in the morning does not interfere with night time sleep, the same activity can interfere with sleep if the time interval from bedtime is too short.

■ **Avoid Caffeinated Drinks Already in the Afternoon Hours**

Caution with caffeine

You should not drink caffeinated beverages after 2 pm. Caffeine stimulates brain activity and thus has a negative effect on sleep. While moderate consumption of caffeine during the day usually does not affect night sleep, excessive and regular consumption can lead to withdrawal symptoms and sleep problems at night. This is true of coffee and black or green tea, as well as cola and stimulant soft drinks. The wakefulness-inducing breakdown products can still be detected in the body up to 14 h after consumption.

■ **Limit Your Nicotine Consumption**

Nicotine stimulates

Apart from the largely known damage caused by tobacco consumption, nicotine has a stimulating effect, just like caffeine. Therefore, stop smoking at least 3 h before going to bed. Nicotine is also a stimulant that can disrupt sleep and interrupt night time sleep due to withdrawal symptoms. Smokers who give up their habit fall asleep faster and wake up less often at night once the withdrawal symptoms are overcome.

■ **Avoid Alcohol Before Bedtime**

Avoid alcohol in the evening

A nightcap disrupts the flow of sleep more than it promotes it and can be responsible for premature morning awakenings. Alcohol lowers brain activity. Drinking alcohol before bed helps you fall asleep at first, but leads to sleep interruptions later in the night, especially worsening the restfulness of sleep the second half of the night. A "nightcap" before falling asleep can cause waking reactions, nightmares, and morning headaches.

- **Do Not Go to Bed Hungry, But Do Not Go to Bed Feeling Full Either**

You should have eaten the last "big meal" 2–3 h before going to bed. If you are still hungry, however, have a small snack before going to bed, so that you do not wake up due to hunger. Dairy products or bananas are ideal for this, as they contain the substance tryptophan, which is beneficial for sleep.

Food and sleep

- **Provide a Comfortable Sleeping Environment**

A comfortable bed and a dark room are important prerequisites for a good night's sleep. A cool but not cold room and fresh air are helpful. If possible, the bedroom should be dedicated exclusively to resting and sleeping. Make sure that you are not disturbed in the bedroom by the telephone or by fellow human beings. Avoid using the bed for anything other than sleeping. You should not be in bed to read, watch TV, eat, work, or even argue with your partner.

Pleasant sleeping environment

- **Relax Before You Go to Bed**

Small personal rituals for falling asleep can help here: a warm bath, a cup of calming tea, light reading, relaxing music, and relaxation exercises (▶ Sect. 8.3 in this chapter).

- **What to Do When Lying Awake in Bed?**

As a general rule, do not go to sleep until you feel tired. Get up if you cannot fall asleep and distract yourself with something to do. If necessary, write down thoughts and worries that run through your mind. Do not fall asleep out of bed. Do not go back to bed until you feel sleepy. Repeat this process as often as necessary if you cannot sleep at night. Do not drive yourself crazy because you cannot fall asleep. Instead, try to accept the situation and enjoy your awake time in a pleasant way and keep yourself busy with other things. Sleep cannot be forced. It usually sets in on its own when we do not "actively want" it to. People who suffer from insomnia should therefore avoid looking at the clock. Many people whose sleep is disturbed sleep better when the time pressure is removed. Hide the alarm clock in the wardrobe, for example, to stop the urge to check the time. And last but not least, get up at your usual time in the morning, even if you feel you have hardly slept at all in the past night.

Sleep cannot be forced

▪ Recreation and Vacation

Vacation enriches our lives

While sleep is our most important passive measure of regeneration, vacation is our most important active measure of recovery. Vacation is often the only time of the year when we can really free ourselves from the constraints and hectic pace of everyday life. On holiday we can regain the energies used up in everyday life, recharge our batteries. We find inner peace and return to our workplaces and everyday lives more resilient and balanced. Holidays also enrich our lives beyond the actual holiday period by providing us with new stimuli, experiences, and impressions. We are positively stimulated by new people, countries, cultures we get to know or by experiencing ourselves in new situations and trying new things. These, at least, are the opportunities that a truly relaxing vacation offers. We should take advantage of these opportunities. For this, it essentially comes down to this:

1. That we plan and design the holiday from the beginning in such a way that it itself is free from hectic, stress and burdensome demands, and
2. That we tailor our holidays as closely as possible to our own personal recreational needs and allow ourselves to be influenced as little as possible by others or by any standards.

How can this succeed?

Which type of holiday is right for me?

▪ Recognize and Take Seriously One's Own Recreational Needs

In order to be able to recover optimally on holiday, we need to know, what we want to recover from, what the previous stress was like. Whether it is a summer or winter holiday, a holiday in the local area or a long-distance trip, an active holiday or lazing on the beach, an extensive sightseeing tour, a city trip or a nature experience, an individual or group trip, organized or on your own, which type of holiday is right for you this year depends solely on your recreational needs and should be a matter of personal choice alone. Therefore, before you worry about the geographical destination and the external organization of the holiday, you should think in detail about your desires and goals that you have for your holiday. Do not let others persuade you to do something that does not correspond to your wishes. And please avoid any thought of prestige or achievement when it comes to your holiday.

▪ Clarify Expectations

When several people go on holiday together, conflicts are often pre-programmed—one person wants to go to the beach and relax other hopes for disco and new contacts, the next wants extensive city walks and museum visits. That is why it is important to clarify with your fellow travellers or with the family what everyone wants to do before the holiday. Only then does the joint and creative search for the type of holiday and the vacation resort follow, where as many of the different wishes as possible can be reconciled.

Sometimes your holiday wishes can't be reconciled. Instead of making lazy compromises, go your separate ways for a few days. Or you can agree on a "patchwork holiday": first, everyone does something for themselves, and then do something together. Or the father does something alone with the children for a few days, while the mother has time for herself, and then there are a few more days of family vacation together. What is needed here is respect for each other's wishes and the courage to find creative, if necessary unconventional solutions. Do not be impressed by prefabricated holiday clichés.

No "lazy" compromises

In general, you should not overload your holiday with expectations, not project onto your holiday all the expectations you have built up or that have been disappointed over the course of the year, for example, for a harmonious and fulfilled partnership, a happy family life. For all the anticipation: stay realistic and do not expect the perfect holiday. Then you can perhaps more easily overlook negative experiences during the holidays (traffic jams, bad weather, unfriendly staff, arguments) instead of getting angry.

Realistic expectations

■ **Slowly Switch to Recovery**

Body and soul need time to switch off on holiday. Physical and mental tension cannot be released at the push of a button. Recovery does not begin immediately after we have closed the office door behind us. Body and soul need a phase of "cool down", of switching off and distancing themselves. Take the time for this. Consciously close your work, clean up your workspace, and prepare it for resuming work after the holiday. Avoid trying to get everything and anything done in the last few days of work before the holiday begins. Do not rush from one appointment to the next until just before you leave, or everyday stress will turn directly into holiday stress. Instead, make a list of unfinished tasks and unsolved problems that you will tackle with renewed vigour after the holiday. This helps to gain distance.

Time for "Cooldown"

Then start your holiday as unhurriedly as possible. Do not set off at the end of a working day, but take at least one day to switch off. Pack in peace and then, when you feel the anticipation inside you, it is the right time to start.

Make yourself clear: If you take the necessary time for this distancing phase, then you will not waste precious vacation days, but lay the foundation for a really relaxing vacation. At most for people whose work is characterized by boredom, underchallenge and too much routine, the motto "Let's get out of here!" applies, because they already have enough distance.

8

■ **Allow Yourself a Sufficiently Long Regeneration Phase**

Refuelling takes time

Only after the distancing phase, when physical and mental tension have been reduced, does the actual regeneration begin, the refuelling. Recovery researchers say that body and soul need at least 3 weeks to recover. This is especially true when you travel to a different time zone or climate. Jet lag and the change to a different climate can also put a strain on body and soul. This is especially true for people under a lot of stress.

■ **Forget Work**

"You can do without me"

Even though it may be difficult at first: stay away from anything that reminds you of your daily work. This applies to technical literature as well as mobile phones and laptops. Switch off your mobile phone! This will also eliminate one of the most common sources of conflict with fellow travellers. Even if it makes you uneasy at first, give yourself the relief of knowing that the shop can run without you if need be. If there is no other way: agree with your company or business partners on certain times when you can be reached, for example, in the morning from 9–10 o'clock. However, it is usually sufficient to check your voicemail once a day.

■ **Come Back and Warm Up**

Warm up slowly

The regeneration phase should not be ended abruptly. What athletes do in the "warm-up phase" before a competition is also important for other activities. Body and mind should be prepared slowly for the new stress. End your holiday period with a day off at home to give your organism time to readjust. Take your time to arrive again. Unpack in peace and get in the mood for the new work week. If you then feel joyful excitement, perhaps even desire for what is to come, then you are truly recovered.

■ **Let the Holiday Linger**

Vacation in everyday life

Has everyday life got you back? Look at your holiday photos at the latest 1 or 2 weeks after your return. In which situations were you particularly happy, in which photos are you laughing? If you look back on your days off and think about which elements you particularly enjoyed, you can plan these specifically for your next holiday. Save the relaxation you gained on holiday for everyday life. For example, start with lighter work tasks after a vacation and continue your vacation habits (reading, exercising, eating in peace) at home.

Questions for Self-reflection: Identifying Recovery Needs

- In which area is recovery particularly important for me this year? Do I feel primarily physically exhausted or more emotionally or mentally drained?
- What kind of holiday would have little or no recreational value for me in my current state of mind? What could I not use at all?
- Do I want to be able to just do nothing, dawdle and hang out this year on vacation?
- Am I looking for inspiring new impressions, new contacts, and encounters?
- Do I have a desire to be physically active?
- Am I dreaming of the deserted island, the bustling resort or immersing myself in a big city?
- What kind of vacation would be the most relaxing for me this year if I did not have to consider anything or anyone?

8.2 Enjoyment in Everyday Life

Whatever you do in your free time, it is crucial for the recreational value that your leisure activities actually create a counterbalance to the stresses of everyday life and work. Leisure activities are truly relaxing when they allow you to unwind and switch off from work, when they are self-determined and evoke positive emotions, fun, and joy in you. Time pressure and performance thinking are usually counterproductive, as is a competitive attitude and prestige thinking. Relaxing leisure activities are more process-oriented than result-oriented. They are determined by the joy not so much of the result as of the activity itself. The focus is not on the purpose of the activity, but on fun, pleasure, and enjoyment. It is also very important that leisure activities are based on voluntariness and not on a sense of obligation. Freeing oneself from the norms and demands and expectations of others is the prerequisite for being able to enjoy leisure time as one's own "free time", as "me time". No longer "I have to do that", but "I treat myself to that" is the motto that stands on the entrance gate to the regenerative counter-world.

As early as the twelfth century, the Cistercian monk Bernard of Clairvaux (1090–1153), one of the most impor-

Free time is free time

tant theologians of the Middle Ages, gave his pastoral advice on this matter. In a treatise dedicated to Pope Eugene III, he urgently exhorts the pope, who was his former monk, not only to be there for others, but also to think of himself:

> » Treat yourself! If you want to be completely there for everyone, I praise your humanity, but only if it is full and real. But how can you be fully and genuinely human if you have lost yourself? You too are a human being. So that your humanity may be all-embracing and perfect, you must have an attentive heart not only for all others, but also for yourself. (...) Yes, he who treats himself badly, to whom can he be good? So remember: treat yourself. I do not say: do this always, I do not say: do this often, but I say: do it again and again.—(Bernard of Clairvaux, important theologian of the Middle Ages, 1090–1153)

■   **Pleasant Experiences: Past and Present**

8

What do I enjoy?

Which specific leisure activities make up your own personal counter-world is, of course, highly individual. Personal preferences, previous experience, and possibilities play an important role here. Whether nature or culture, whether sport or music, whether dance or pottery—the decisive factor is that you experience joy, pleasure, and leisure in the process and, above all, that you allow yourself your free time without a guilty conscience. However, I often meet people who no longer know what it could be that could give them fun and joy, what they could experience as pleasant, relaxing, and restful. They are already in the permanent stress-depression spiral. Due to the ongoing stress of everyday life, access to positive experiences has literally been buried. Life has become more and more narrowed down to dealing with the demands of work and everyday life. Here it can be helpful to think back to earlier times—even in the distant past if necessary—and to activities that gave pleasure at that time (box "To think further" and checklist "Pleasant experiences" in ◘ Fig. 8.2).

■   **To Think Further**
—   What leisure activities did I enjoy in the past?
—   What was good for me?
—   What things or activities allowed me to really switch off?

When you are dealing with these questions, you might also look into old photo albums or take mementos (the old hiking shoes, piano notes, the tennis racket, the cookbook, travel souvenirs ...) in your hand. This helps to jog your memory and bring it to life.

List of pleasant experiences						
The following list contains a number of activities that many people experience as pleasant and relaxing. For each activity, please indicate how much you enjoy doing it and how often you do it. The list is not exhaustive. If you can think of other possibilities, please write them on the blank lines.						
What?	**How much do you like?**			**How often?**		
	Not	**something**	**very**	**never**	**rarely**	**often**
1. Contact and Socializing						
Visiting friends/acquaintances/relatives	☹	😐	☺	☹	😐	☺
Invite friends/acquaintances/relatives	☹	😐	☺	☹	😐	☺
Playing with children	☹	😐	☺	☹	😐	☺
Visiting a pub	☹	😐	☺	☹	😐	☺
Making phone calls, chatting	☹	😐	☺	☹	😐	☺
Going dancing	☹	😐	☺	☹	😐	☺
Going on trips with family/friends or acquaintances	☹	😐	☺	☹	😐	☺
Playing board games	☹	😐	☺	☹	😐	☺
Participating in a club (bowling club, choir, chess club, etc.)	☹	😐	☺	☹	😐	☺
What else comes to mind:						
–	☹	😐	☺	☹	😐	☺
–	☹	😐	☺	☹	😐	☺
2. Hobbies						
Taking photos/films	☹	😐	☺	☹	😐	☺
Collecting stamps/coins	☹	😐	☺	☹	😐	☺
Growing plants	☹	😐	☺	☹	😐	☺
Painting/Drawing	☹	😐	☺	☹	😐	☺

Fig. 8.2 List of pleasant experiences

What?	How much?			How often?		
	Not	**something**	**very**	**never**	**rarely**	**often**
Pottery	☹	😐	☺	☹	😐	☺
Crafts/Handicrafts	☹	😐	☺	☹	😐	☺
Playing a musical instrument	☹	😐	☺	☹	😐	☺
Gardening	☹	😐	☺	☹	😐	☺
Singing	☹	😐	☺	☹	😐	☺
Cooking something special	☹	😐	☺	☹	😐	☺
Solving puzzles/riddles	☹	😐	☺	☹	😐	☺
Technical games (train, computer…)	☹	😐	☺	☹	😐	☺
DIY	☹	😐	☺	☹	😐	☺
What else comes to mind:						
–	☹	😐	☺	☹	😐	☺
–	☹	😐	☺	☹	😐	☺
3. Culture and Education						
Going to a concert	☹	😐	☺	☹	😐	☺
Going to the theatre	☹	😐	☺	☹	😐	☺
Going to the cinema	☹	😐	☺	☹	😐	☺
Listening to a lecture	☹	😐	☺	☹	😐	☺
Visiting exhibitions/museums	☹	😐	☺	☹	😐	☺
Reading a good book	☹	😐	☺	☹	😐	☺
Taking a course	☹	😐	☺	☹	😐	☺
Learn a foreign language	☹	😐	☺	☹	😐	☺
What else comes to mind						
–	☹	😐	☺	☹	😐	☺
–	☹	😐	☺	☹	😐	☺

◘ Fig. 8.2 (continued)

What?	How much?			How often?		
	Not	**Something**	**Very**	**Never**	**Rarely**	**Often**
4. Sports and Exercise						
Walking/hiking	☹	😐	☺	☹	😐	☺
Forest running/jogging	☹	😐	☺	☹	😐	☺
Tennis	☹	😐	☺	☹	😐	☺
Table tennis	☹	😐	☺	☹	😐	☺
Swimming	☹	😐	☺	☹	😐	☺
Cycling	☹	😐	☺	☹	😐	☺
Winter sports (ski hiking, downhill ski, snowboard...)	☹	😐	☺	☹	😐	☺
Ball sports	☹	😐	☺	☹	😐	☺
Gymnastics/aerobics/Pilates etc.	☹	😐	☺	☹	😐	☺
Water sports (sailing, rowing, canoeing...)	☹	😐	☺	☹	😐	☺
Strength training	☹	😐	☺	☹	😐	☺
What else comes to mind:						
–	☹	😐	☺	☹	😐	☺
–	☹	😐	☺	☹	😐	☺
5. Nature experiences and "Passivities"						
Lying in the grass	☹	😐	☺	☹	😐	☺
Watching animals (e.g. birds)	☹	😐	☺	☹	😐	☺
Walking barefoot	☹	😐	☺	☹	😐	☺
Picking flowers (e.g. in a meadow)	☹	😐	☺	☹	😐	☺
Sitting in the sun	☹	😐	☺	☹	😐	☺
Picking herbs, mushrooms etc.	☹	😐	☺	☹	😐	☺
Enjoying a beautiful view	☹	😐	☺	☹	😐	☺

◘ **Fig. 8.2** (continued)

Was?	How much?			How often?		
	Not	Something	Very	Never	Rarely	Often
Sitting by the stove/looking into the fire	☹	😐	☺	☹	😐	☺
Sauna	☹	😐	☺	☹	😐	☺
Sunrise, sunset, stars, Cloud watching	☹	😐	☺	☹	😐	☺
Fishing	☹	😐	☺	☹	😐	☺
Wading in the water	☹	😐	☺	☹	😐	☺
Drinking a good cup of tea/coffee	☹	😐	☺	☹	😐	☺
Listening to music	☹	😐	☺	☹	😐	☺
Taking a bath	☹	😐	☺	☹	😐	☺
Getting a massage	☹	😐	☺	☹	😐	☺
Sitting in a pavement café	☹	😐	☺	☹	😐	☺
What else comes to mind:						
–	☹	😐	☺	☹	😐	☺
–	☹	😐	☺	☹	😐	☺

Evaluation:
Now please look at the completed sheet again: Are there any activities or "passivities" that you enjoy but rarely or never experience? Have you perhaps come across things that you would have liked to do but have always postponed? Are there activities that you used to enjoy doing and that you would like take up again? Please write down on this sheet the pleasant things you would like to do in the next few weeks to compensate for your stress.

_____

_____

_____

_____

◻ **Fig. 8.2**   (continued)

The Eight Rules of Enjoyment

Can you learn to enjoy? In their therapeutic work with depressive patients, the two psychotherapists Rainer Lutz and Eva Koppenhöfer from the Psychosomatic Specialist Clinic in Bad Dürckheim have repeatedly observed that these patients, even when they perform activities that are usually fun or enjoyable for other people, cannot really take pleasure in them. Yes, worse still, often the depressive moods worsen by this experience. People who are permanently stressed and burnt out also experience something similar. They can no longer be happy or enjoy themselves. Lutz and Koppenhöfer have drawn the conclusion that it is not enough to motivate these people to become active again, but that they first have to learn to enjoy again. To this end, they have developed a "Little School of Enjoyment". Since enjoyment in everyday life is also a very important source of compensation for stressful situations for stress-ridden people, I will give the most important rules of enjoyment in the following in a slightly modified form. Perhaps you, will find here valuable tips and suggestions for the design of your personal everyday enjoyment.

Enjoyment has to be learned

Treat Yourself to Pleasure

Many people have inhibitions, a guilty conscience or feel ashamed when they do something good for themselves. It is as if they are not entitled to enjoyment or the joy of life. Perhaps because they were forbidden to do so by their parents in their childhood, they cannot allow themselves to enjoy themselves today. Here it is important to get aware of prohibitions of enjoyment that have become unnecessary and to overcome them.

Little school of enjoyment

> I would have wanted to do it, but I didn't dare to be allowed.—
> (Karl Valentin, comedian and writer, 1882–1948)

Take Time to Enjoy

This sounds banal but it is a very important prerequisite for enjoyment. Enjoyment is not possible under time pressure— but sometimes a moment is enough.

Enjoy Consciously

If you do many things at the same time, you will hardly be able to enjoy them. If you want to experience pleasure, then you have to switch off the other activities and concentrate completely on this. Enjoyment is not something you can do on the side. Constantly thinking about future or past tasks often obscures your view of the pleasurable. Enjoyment takes place in the present.

8

> Do you want to wander on and on? See, the good is so close!
> Only learn to grasp happiness, for happiness is always there.—
> (Johann Wolfgang von Goethe, 1749–1832)

■ **School Your Senses for Pleasure**

Enjoyment presupposes a finely differentiated sensory perception that has been formed through experience. Enjoyment depends on the perception of nuances. It is important here to sharpen one's own senses.

■ **Enjoy in Your Own Way**

As the saying goes: "What's one man's owl is another man's nightingale". Enjoyment means something different for everyone. Here it is important to find out what is good for you and—just as important—what is not good for you and what is good for you when.

■ **Enjoy Rather Little, but Properly**

A popular misconception about enjoyment is that the person who consumes more enjoys more. However, it is not the quantity but the quality that is decisive for enjoyment. Too much has a satiating and boring effect in the long run. We therefore advocate limiting oneself, not out of stinginess or false modesty, but in order to treat oneself to the best in each case.

■ **Planning Creates Anticipation**

There is a saying that one should celebrate the festivities as they fall. The coincidental, spontaneous, unexpected often brings a very special pleasure. However, it does not seem favourable to leave enjoyment to chance alone. In everyday life, it will often be necessary to plan pleasant experiences, i.e. to allocate the time for them, to make the appropriate preparations, to arrange appointments, and so on. This has the additional pleasant effect of allowing you to look forward to the forthcoming pleasurable event for some time in advance.

■ **Enjoy the Little Things in Everyday Life**

The little happiness
Pleasure is not always necessarily something quite extraordinary. Quite a few people miss out on the small happiness while they wait in vain for the big one. It is important to find pleasure in normal everyday life—in small occurrences and everyday activities. Those who keep themselves inwardly open to this in everyday life can discover a multitude of sources for pleasant experiences especially in everyday life. Perceiving everyday things from a different, non-purposeful point of view can bring unexpected pleasures.

» Happiness often comes from paying attention to small things, unhappiness often comes from neglecting small things.— (Wilhelm Busch, 1832–1908)

Enjoyment in Everyday Life: Positive Daily Review
In the coming days, consciously pay attention to beautiful things in your everyday life. Look at what brings you joy, what you find pleasant, and what you can enjoy. These can be special events, such as the rare visit of good friends or, for example, a visit to the theatre. But even more important are the small everyday pleasures, such as the pleasant feeling on your skin after your morning shower, or a beautiful sunset you have watched, or the pleasant smell of freshly ground coffee. Take a few minutes each day to review your day in a positive way. Visualize what you experienced as pleasant that day.

8.3 Relax and Let Go

The rhythmic alternation between tension and relaxation is an essential characteristic of the living. Just think of the rhythm of breathing with its alternation of inspiration and expiration or the lively pulsation of the heart with its alternation of contraction and expansion. Here tension and relaxation form a dynamic unity like the sunny and shady sides of a mountain. One exists only as a counterpart of the other. Strong tension tires and leads to a natural relaxation. Relaxation rebuilds energy reserves, making new tension possible. The aim of relaxation training is to support and promote such a lively alternation between tension and relaxation, and especially to get it going again where it is out of sync or completely interrupted due to long-lasting or recurring stresses.

Alternation of tension and relaxation

■ **Relaxation Training: How It Works and What It Does**
The ability to relax physically and switch off mentally is a fundamental way of coping with stress. Basically, everyone has this ability and—and this is the good news—it can be trained. What is required—as with the training of any other skill—is regular practice. Regular practice over a period of three to 4 months is the key to success. By then, most people have trained their ability to relax to such an extent that they can use it profitably in or before difficult situations. The following experiences are significant on the way there:

Relaxation can be trained

8

■ Sense Tension

The path to relaxation

Many people have lost the sense for physical tension processes. They only notice them when symptoms of excessive tension (e.g. headaches and neck pain, stomach complaints, eye pressure, sleep disorders, etc.) have already set in. The first aim and effect of relaxation training are therefore often to sharpen our perception of tension sensations so that we can take countermeasures as early as possible. We perceive physical signals of tension more sensitively.

■ Experience the Change from Tension to Relaxation

In the course of relaxation training, we then become more and more aware of the difference between states of tension and relaxation. We will experience how pleasant feelings of relaxation gradually begin to spread through our body as the tension subsides. And we will gradually learn to consciously bring about this "switch" from tension to relaxation.

■ Enjoy Relaxation

Inner restlessness and nervousness gradually decrease, and we become more and more successful in maintaining a pleasant, deep state of relaxation over a limited period of time and experiencing it with pleasure. We memorize the sensations of relaxation as deeply as possible in order to be able to recall them in normal everyday life.

■ Bringing Relaxation into Everyday Life

The ultimate goal is to enable us to use the trained relaxation skills in everyday situations. We learn how to experience pleasant feelings of relaxation not only during the special relaxation exercises in the "quiet chamber", so to speak, but how to carry them out into normal everyday life.

Stress complaints decrease

The positive health effects that can be achieved through relaxation training have been proven beyond doubt in numerous scientific studies. Regular relaxation exercises lead to a reduction in physical tension and subsequently to an alleviation of many stress-related physical complaints, such as sleep disorders, headaches, circulatory disorders, and heart complaints. People who start with relaxation training report already after the first exercises that they feel their own body and thus themselves better again. They feel more centred again, connected to their own centre. People who regularly perform relaxation exercises also report a feeling of increasing mental relaxation, a deep experience of calm and serenity, as well as a feeling of recovery and mental freshness immediately after the exercises. In the longer term, relaxation training can also contribute to a higher degree of self-confidence and a reduction in anxious and depressed moods.

■ **Methods of Relaxation Training**

Various training methods have been developed to train the ability to relax. In German-speaking countries, these include in particular autogenic training (AT), which was founded by the Berlin physician Johannes Heinrich Schultz in the 1920s, and progressive muscle relaxation (PMR) according to Edmund Jacobson.

There is extensive practical experience and scientific evidence of effectiveness for both methods. Both methods also have in common that they work without external aids, such as audio cassettes or CDs, and aim at the trainees learning to create the state of relaxation out of themselves (= autogenous). In my experience, PMR has the advantage over AT that it leads to initial successes more quickly, at least for most people, and thus motivates them to continue practicing. This is especially true for permanently stressed people with a high basic tension. They often find a quick and easy access to first relaxation experiences with PMR. Therefore, I will describe the method of PMR in more detail in the following.

■ **Progressive Muscle Relaxation (PMR)**

The method was developed in the 1930s by the American physician and neurophysiologist Edmund Jacobson. Jacobson assumed that every mental tension is also expressed in muscular tension. Therefore, a gradual release of mental tension should be possible through progressive muscular relaxation. Based on this basic idea, he developed a system of exercises for the differentiated relaxation of the entire muscular system.

The **basic principle of** the method is very simple (▣ Fig. 8.3). It consists of alternating between tension and subsequent relaxation of individual muscle groups. To do this, individual muscles are first consciously tensed. The tension is held briefly and then released and relaxed again with the exhalation. Concentrate on the sensations of relaxation in the relevant muscle areas and deepen the relaxation with each exhalation.

So with PMR you learn to relax some major muscle groups of your body in a specific order, first tensing and then relaxing these muscle groups, while at the same time paying very concentrated and careful attention to the sensations that occur in your muscles as you do so. With some practice, you will come to lower your muscle tension well below normal tension levels, whenever you want and whenever you need.

Learning to relax is similar to learning other skills, such as swimming, driving, or playing the piano. You need practice, concentration, and commitment to do it. This means that you need to take time, time for yourself. There is nothing mysterious about the method either, you do not have to believe in it.

Relaxation methods

PMR basic principle

Draw attention to the
respective body region

Tense the muscles

Hold the tension briefly (approx. 5-7 sec.)
while continuing to breathe.

With the exhale release tension
and relax (30-45 sec.)

◘ Fig. 8.3   Basic principle of progressive muscle relaxation (PMR)

You just have to practice. Even Erich Kästner knew: "There is nothing good unless you do it!".

Practice regularly

With a little practice, you will notice that by relaxing the muscles, other signs of physical restlessness and agitation, such as palpitations, sweating, trembling decrease or disappear, that you feel much calmer and more relaxed overall. With muscle relaxation you therefore have a technique at hand with which you can reduce physical and mental tension and nervousness and cope with everyday stressful situations more calmly.

If you would like to start with relaxation training, then please take the following practical tips to heart. For lasting training success, it is advisable to carry out the training under professional guidance. Appropriate courses are offered by adult education centres, health insurance companies, and the like.

▪ **Practical Tips: What Matters When Practicing**

Tense and Relax

By tensing a group of muscles and then releasing the resulting tension with the exhale, you allow those muscles to relax well below their normal tension level. The effect is similar to a pendulum hanging down motionless. If we want it to swing strongly to the left ("relaxation") , we could push it strongly in that direction. However, it would be easier to first pull it completely in the opposite direction ("tension") and then let it fall. It will swing beyond vertical in the desired direction. Tightening the muscles before relaxing is like helping ourselves to a "flying start" into deep relaxation. At the same time, tensing should not exceed 5–7 s, so as not to cramp the muscles. Continue to breathe normally while tensing and please do not hold your breath. After relaxing a muscle group, you should take about 30 s to let the relaxation take effect.

- ■ **The Muscle Groups**

▢ Table 8.1 shows which muscle groups you can tense and how. As you can see, the complete exercise consists of four exercise parts, each with four muscle groups. Start with the first exercise part and then add another exercise part from exercise week to exercise week. After 4 weeks of practice, you will have mastered the complete exercise, with which you can relax all the major muscle groups of your body.

How to practice with success

▢ **Table 8.1** Progressive muscle relaxation—how to tense the muscles

1. Exercise part: hands, and arms	
(1) Dominant hand and forearm	Clench your fist
(2) Dominant upper arm	Bend elbow (with open hand)
(3) Non-dominant hand and forearm	Clench your fist
(4) Non-dominant upper arm	Bend elbow (with open hand)
2. Exercise part: feet, legs, buttocks	
(5) Feet	Dig one's toes in *or* Spread your toes
(6) Lower leg	Lift heels off the floor (Caution: If you have a tendency to calf cramps, lift heels only slightly!)
(7) Thigh	Press heels into floor and lift toes off floor
(8) Buttocks	Squeeze the buttocks
3. Exercise part: head and face	
(9) Forehead and scalp	Raise eyebrows and at the same time put the forehead in horizontal folds *or* Eyebrows pull together so that on the forehead formed deep vertical wrinkles ("frown lines")

(continued)

8

☐ **Table 8.1** (continued)	
(10) Eyes and upper cheek area	Squint your eyes and pull your nose up ("wrinkle").
(11) Lower cheek area, jaw, mouth	Clench your teeth, press your lips together, press your tongue up against the roof of your mouth.
(12) Neck and throat	Pull head in slightly and push back *or* Pull head forward onto chest *or* Turn head slightly to the right (or left), chin pointing to the right (or left) shoulder. *or* Tilt the head face down towards the right (or left) shoulder ("put the ear on the shoulder").
4. Exercise part: shoulders, back, chest, abdomen	
(13) Shoulders and upper back	Raise shoulders ("up to the ears") *or* Press shoulder blades backwards (as if the tips of the shoulder blades wanted to touch each other) *or* Pull shoulders forward in front of chest.
(14) Breast	Inhale deeply and hold your breath briefly, tensing the chest muscles.
(15) Lower back	Make a slight hollow back by tilting the pelvis forward *or* Bend the torso forward.
(16) Belly	Make belly hard (as if you want to catch a light blow) *or* Retract abdominal wall *or* Abdomen bulging outward

■ **Pay Attention to Sensations**

Another advantage of the technique of first creating tension and then relaxing is that the contrast makes it easier for you to recognize and distinguish between the sensations associated with tension and relaxation. When you tense a muscle group, you feel the muscles harden and contract. Always pay close attention to these sensations as you tense. When you then relax the muscle group, that is release all tension at the same time, these sensations disappear, and pleasant feelings of relaxation take their place. These can be quite different from person to person. Some people feel warmth flowing into their muscles or a pleasant tingling sensation, others feel heaviness or weightlessness. It is only important that you pay close attention to these sensations during relaxation, feel them and thus allow the relaxation to become deeper and deeper.

■ **Breathe Correctly**

When tensing the muscles, you should continue to breathe normally, that is do not hold your breath. When the tension is released, exhale deeply. Otherwise, you should not pay any further attention to your breathing or even try to control it. During the exercise, you will come to calm and relaxed breathing all by yourself.

■ **Digressive Thoughts**

You will find that it is not easy to concentrate only on yourself or on the muscle relaxation. Your attention will be distracted more often by sounds, other bodily sensations, or wandering thoughts. This is normal and should not worry you. If you find that you have become distracted, accept it calmly, and then return your attention to your body. So do not think about it any further, just continue with the exercise. It often helps to give yourself the instructions for the exercise by speaking inwardly, and also to comment inwardly on the sensations that occur as you relax. For example, "...exhale and relax. Let out all tension and focus entirely on the sensations that occur as the muscles relax. Notice how they become softer and more relaxed...", etc.

■ **Time**

Practice at least once a day, and time it so that you have 20 min to start with, during which you will not be disturbed and will not feel under time pressure. These minutes should therefore be completely at your disposal for relaxation.

■ **External Environment**

Especially at the beginning of the training, it is particularly important that you are not distracted and disturbed in your concentration during the practice. A quiet, possibly darkened room is therefore ideal. Make sure that you are not interrupted by people or pets in the room or by the ringing of the telephone or doorbell.

■ **Seating**

The seating should be such that no effort is required for posture. A well-upholstered chair in which you can comfortably lean or rest your head, neck, back, and arms is ideal. The feet should have good contact with the floor.

■ Clothes

Make sure that you are not restricted in your freedom of movement and ability to concentrate by constricting clothing (jacket, tie, belt, uncomfortable shoes, etc.) or glasses, contact lenses, watches, etc. during the exercise. Take them off beforehand.

■ Basic Position

Before you start the relaxation exercises, you should take a minute to make sure that you are really comfortable and relaxed and prepare yourself to relax.

When you practice sitting, make sure your feet are comfortable, your legs are relaxed, you can lean anywhere properly, you can find a comfortable position for your head, your shoulders are hanging down loosely, and your hands and forearms are relaxed on the backrest or in your lap.

Of course, you can also practice lying down. Lie on your back with your arms slightly bent, your legs stretched out next to each other and your feet pointing outwards. You may find it more comfortable to place a pillow or roll on the back of your neck, back or the back of your knees. Try out the position that is most comfortable for you.

■ Clear Start

— From the beginning, please get into the habit of starting each relaxation exercise with a little ritual. This starting ritual looks like this:

1. You consciously decide you want to do the exercise now and say to yourself, "Now I'm going to relax."
2. You consciously assume your relaxation position (sit with your buttocks on the entire seat and lean your back against it, place your feet firmly on the floor, place your hands on your thighs, and let your shoulders fall).
3. You consciously turn your attention inwards, to your body, and close your eyes.

■ Clear End

When you have relaxed all the main muscle groups, try to maintain and enjoy the pleasant state of relaxation for a few minutes. To do this, you can go through the individual muscle groups again in your mind and feel the degree of your relaxation or simply remain relaxed and indulge in a pleasant imagination. Then tell yourself that you want to end the relaxation. Take your time doing this. Clench your hands into fists, stretch, and loll, take a few deep breaths and then open your eyes. This will bring the body back to the waking state after relaxation, much like sleeping. This withdrawal of relaxation

□ Table 8.2   Progressive muscle relaxation—short form

(1) Arms:	Clench both hands into fists and bend elbows
(2) Head:	Draw eyebrows together, wrinkle your nose, clench your teeth and lips, pull your head in slightly, and push it back
(3) Hull:	Squeeze shoulders back down, slightly hollow back, and make abdominal wall hard
(4) Legs:	Press both heels to the floor, raise toes, tense lower leg, thigh, and gluteal muscles

should take place after each exercise. Only if you practice in bed in the evening immediately before sleeping, do **not** take back the relaxation. Otherwise you may feel fresh and rested and therefore not be able to sleep in the following hours. If you do not take back the relaxation in bed, you will fall asleep better.

■ **Shortening the Relaxation Exercise**

If you have trained PMR in the manner described over a period of 3–4 weeks, then you have usually mastered the method so well that you can begin to shorten the exercise. For this purpose, you combine the individual muscles into groups, which you then simultaneously first tense and then relax. According to the four exercise parts of the long form, you can shorten the exercise to four muscle groups. For details of how to tense the muscle groups, please refer to □ Table 8.2.

PMR short form

■ **Short Exercises for Everyday Life**

For intermediate relaxation in everyday life, you can use short exercises in which only individual muscles and muscle groups are tensed and then relaxed. You will find instructions for two short exercises that have proved successful in practice in the boxes "King Kong exercise" and "Quasimodo exercise". The effect of such short exercises will be stronger the more intense you have previously trained your ability to relax by means of the longer exercises.

Exercise "King Kong"

This exercise is mainly used to relax the shoulders, arms, and hands. For many people, it is an effective short-term way to reduce inner tension. The exercise can be performed while sitting or standing. To perform the exercise, proceed as follows:

Keep your arms bent in front of your chest. The elbows are at shoulder height, and the hands are clenched into fists. Close your eyes and continue breathing throughout the exercise. Do not hold your breath. Vigorously tense all arm and upper body muscles. Fists, forearms, upper arms, shoulders, and chest—now. Hold the tension for a moment, continue breathing—and with the next exhale, lower your arms and relax. Let your arms hang loosely at your sides. If you feel comfortable, you can also let your head hang forward. Feel the relaxation spreading through your upper body. In your hands, in your forearms, in your upper arms. The shoulders also relax and the chest muscles. Breathe calmly and evenly …

Now clench your hands into fists, breathe deeply, and turn your attention back outwards. (Adapted from Brechtel 1994)

8

Exercise "Quasimodo"

This exercise is mainly for relaxing the neck muscles. It is also helpful for emerging headaches, declining concentration and screen work. The exercise can be performed while sitting or standing. To perform the exercise, proceed as follows:

Stand (or sit) upright with your head straight. Pull your shoulders all the way up. As if you want to touch your earlobes with them. Now push your head back without turning your face towards the ceiling. Push the head back, against the cushion that has formed on the back of your neck. Now press the back of the head and the neck cushion together firmly. Continue to breathe calmly and evenly. Feel the tension in your shoulders and neck, all the way down your back …

And with the next exhale, loosely drop your head and shoulders. Drop your head onto your chest until your chin touches your chest and breathe calmly and evenly. Feel the relaxation in your shoulders, neck, and arms …

Now clench your hands into fists, breathe deeply and turn your attention back outwards. (Adapted from Brechtel, 1994)

■ **Excursus: On the Nature of Relaxation**

Centring attention instead of scattering it

Many of the possibilities for relaxation offered in our culture are based on distraction, on the diversion of attention. Attention is thereby turned outward. Just think of the oversized offer of electronic entertainment media. Of course, television can help to switch off from stressful thoughts, everyday worries, or unpleasant feelings. However, the effect usually does not last long. Often the inner restlessness returns all the stronger afterwards. It is not uncommon to be left with a stale feeling of inner emptiness after an evening of television, during which one has zapped through the various programs. The contact with one's own self has been lost, one no longer feels oneself. Thus, what constantly happens in the hectic pace of everyday life is not cancelled here, but only continued, namely that one loses contact with oneself, one's own centre. Psychological relaxation methods are therefore not about distraction and diversion, but about the collection and centring of attention. The attention, which in everyday life is directed towards external stimuli, is now turned inwards, towards one's own self, towards one's own body. This turning of the attention inwards is unusual at first and can even be frightening. The heartbeat, the breath, the pulsation of the blood in the veins, sounds in the stomach and intestines, which normally lie in the shadows of attention, now become conscious. Inner restlessness, circling, or fluttering thoughts become more noticeable. At first, all of this can be more disconcerting than relaxing, and can lead to the desire to distract oneself. With increasing practice, however, it becomes easier and easier to concentrate on oneself with calmness and composure. This is the first important step on the way to physical and mental relaxation.

- **Concentration Without Effort**

Relaxation, however, requires not only an inward turn, but also a very specific form of attention. Two forms of attention can be distinguished: active, tense, goal-oriented concentration. It is concerned with the achievement of a goal, directed towards an object or problem, performance-oriented and controlled by the mind. It is the attention of the actor. In contrast, the second form of attention is more passive, free-floating, flitting; it is observing, registering. It is the attention of the spectator and is also called concentration without effort. Relaxation is about this second, the floating, as it were, form of attention. This, by the way, is not to be confused with sleepiness. It often happens that people who start with relaxation training fall asleep during the first exercises and are quite happy about it, for example, because they have suffered from difficulties in falling asleep up to now. But this is only a transitional stage. In the long term, the aim is to achieve a state of "relaxed alertness", which is characterized by physical relaxation combined with mental alertness. Incidentally, such a state can be detected by characteristic brain wave activity, as EEG studies have shown in people who practiced autogenic training over a longer period of time.

Relaxed alertness

8

■ **Relaxation Cannot Be Forced**

Relaxation means being able to let go

We have emphasized how important concentration and regular practice are for the success of the training. However, being able to relax requires something more, namely: being able to let go, to take time for yourself and to be patient with yourself when things do not go so well. Many of you will also know the experience that just when you desperately want to fall asleep, sleep does not happen. It is only when you give up the intention to sleep and let go of the anger and worry about not getting enough sleep that sleep suddenly comes. It is quite similar with relaxation. It, too, cannot be achieved by any conscious effort of will, no matter how great. Think, for example, of searching for a word, which one finds only when one is no longer frantically trying to find it. Particularly effortful practitioners who use their "whole will", or those who think one can achieve everything with the will, fail. One cannot eliminate tension, cramp (and the phenomena that go with it) with the will—and certainly not release them; for will is tension. On the path of relaxation, there is therefore at the very beginning—and always anew—the necessity to let go of the conscious will, the intention to want to actively influence, control, manage things, in favour of a more perceiving, recording and surrendering attitude.

8.4 Doing Sport and Getting More Exercise in Everyday Life

Sport promotes mental well-being

Physical activity is a good way to protect the organism from the damaging effects of chronic stress. Physical activity, like fight-or-flight behaviour, uses up the energy made available under stress and increases one's resistance to strain. Sport promotes mental well-being and helps to gain distance. The mind is cleared, thoughts come to rest. Sport promotes self-confidence and the confidence to succeed. In a nutshell: Sport is a highly effective stress killer!

■ **Lack of Exercise: A Danger to Health**

Risk factor lack of exercise

Technical progress has radically changed people's lives over the last 100 years. Machines, cars, elevators, escalators, and lawn mowers—to name just a few examples—have made more and more physical work easier for us or taken it away completely. Whereas our grandparents and even our parents often still had to perform heavy physical work and, for example, regularly walked long distances, many people today spend most of the day sitting: in the car or on public transport, in the office, in front of the computer or in meetings, on the sofa at home in front of the television. Life has become more comfortable and pleasant. What is wrong with that? While technical development continues to advance, the human body is still largely comparable to that of prehistoric man, who was at home in the vast savannahs of North Africa. This human body is programmed to move. The human body functions fundamentally different than a machine, which wears out through frequent use. The human body loses its efficiency and becomes susceptible to disease precisely when it is not sufficiently stressed. The results of many scientific studies show more and more clearly that lack of exercise:

- Can lead to obesity,
- Makes the heart work at high speed even in peace,
- Increases the blood pressure,
- Can lead to varicose veins because the blood "pools" in the veins,
- Can contribute to the slackening of certain muscle groups and on the other hand to the cramping of other muscle groups,
- Results in postural weaknesses,
- Can lead to excessive bone loss (osteoporosis),
- Makes the blood sugar rise,
- Makes more susceptible to viral diseases (colds, flu),
- Can promote signs of wear and tear on joints (hips, knees) and intervertebral discs,
- Accelerates aging processes,
- Increases depressive and anxious moods.

Many diseases and ailments that have been considered normal and unavoidable signs of wear and tear of aging are actually due to years of lack of exercise.

- **Reduce Stress Through Exercise**

The positive physical effects of regular physical activity have been documented in numerous scientific studies. Many scientific studies have also shown that in particular endurance sport is associated with increased mental well-being and positive changes in depressive and anxious moods. Thus, regular physical activity contributes significantly to

Positive effects of sport

- Lower blood pressure,
- Lower blood fat and blood sugar levels,
- Strengthen the heart muscle,
- Increase the oxygen-carrying capacity of the lungs,
- Increase resistance, especially against colds,
- Improve the depth and quality of sleep,
- Increase well-being and joie de vivre,
- Alleviate anxiety and depression,
- Increase self-esteem.

> **Important**
> Sports physicians and exercise scientists recommend two ways
> to increase physical activity that provides health benefits:
> — Path 1: Bring more movement into everyday life.
> — Way 2: Exercise regularly.

■ **Path 1: Bringing More Physical Activity into Everyday Life**

Even moderate-intensity physical activities that are common
in everyday life can improve your fitness and help balance
stress. Examples of such activities are:
— Gardening,
— Walking briskly,
— Riding a bike,
— Climbing stairs,
— Shovel snow or sweep leaves.

Just 10 min of exercise promotes health

Such physical activities have health benefits if you do them
daily if possible, but at least 5 days a week for 30 min or more
at a time. The good news is that it is not necessary to be physically active for 30 min at a time. Even several shorter periods of physical activity per day will provide health benefits.
However, an activity duration of 10 min should not be fallen
short of.

Any regular physical activity, which at least leads to an
acceleration of breathing and is performed for at least 10 min,
already promotes health.

Tips: How to get exercise in your everyday life

Here are some practical tips on how you can bring more
physical activity into your everyday life:

■ **Combine Necessary Activities in Everyday Life with
Exercise!**

This is a low-impact way to make your everyday life more
physically active. Think about which of the activities in your
everyday life you could do in a way that makes you move more.
Look specifically for opportunities for physical activity in your
everyday life. Examples include:
— I do not take the bus to work anymore, I walk or ride my
bike.
— I do not use the elevator anymore; I climb the stairs.
— I do minor shopping and errands on foot or by bike.
— When we go on outings with the family, we drive less and
instead take shorter walks or go to the swimming pool.
— When gardening, I use my muscles instead of machines
(lawn mower, hedge trimmer, leaf vacuum, etc.).

■ **Consciously Increase the Duration and Intensity of Physical Activities in Your Everyday Life!**

This option also does not require any special effort. You just need to pay close attention to physical activities that you are already doing. And then consciously extend or strengthen these activities. Examples are:

— When I am walking, I consciously take a step faster.
— When climbing stairs, I take two steps at a time.
— I take fewer breaks when I am gardening.
— In the evening, I walk the dog longer.
— I get off a stop (or two) early and walk the rest.

■ **Schedule Regular Exercise Breaks!**

This option requires a little more effort and planning. It involves deliberately scheduling times of at least 10 min in your daily routine where you engage in moderate physical activity. Examples of this are:

— In the morning before breakfast, do gymnastics for 10 min.
— Leave the office during lunch break and take a short brisk walk.
— In the evening, before going to bed, get out into the fresh air and take a long walk.

> **Observe and Reflect: Bringing More Physical Activity into Everyday Life**
> Go through the usual course of a normal day in your everyday life in your mind and systematically look for opportunities for more physical activity.

■ **Way 2: Exercise Regularly**

The highest benefit for fitness and stress balance brings regular sports activity. Endurance sports as jogging, brisk walking hiking, fast cycling, swimming, and cross-country skiing are particularly beneficial. Endurance sports are sports in which the same movement is repeated over a long period of time. The greater the muscle mass used, the more your circulation and metabolism are taxed. Your body gradually adapts to this increased demand. For example, your heart begins to work more economically. This means that it needs less strength for the same performance and recovers more quickly. This happens through increased blood flow, improved metabolism, and strengthening of the heart muscle.

Regular sports activity

The rhythmic movement during endurance sports relieves mental stress and promotes well-being. Often you have the feeling that the movement happens by itself. The thoughts get free run and little by little the head becomes free.

If you want to start exercising, please follow these tips!

Note before the sport

■ **Beware of Excessive Ambition!**

It is very important that you do the sport for the fun of the movement and with joy in your body. Excessive ambition is out of place here. Listen carefully to your body and pay attention to the signals of your body.

■ **Which Sporting Activity Is Best for Me?**

Simply put, the best physical activity for you is the one you will actually do. What type of physical activity would you enjoy the most? In what kind of environment would you prefer to do physical activity? Do you prefer to exercise indoors or outdoors? Would you prefer to exercise alone or with others? If you are unsure whether a particular sport is right for you, consult a sports doctor if necessary.

■ **Play It Safe!**

Seek medical advice

Exercising regularly can change your life for the better. However, you should not take any unnecessary risks. To be on the safe side, you should seek medical advice **beforehand,** if necessary, if you are

- Older than 35 years,
- Have not exercised regularly during the last 5 years and/or have had a predominantly sedentary lifestyle,
- Overweight,
- A smoker,
- Suffer from diabetes,
- Have high cholesterol or high blood pressure,
- Are recovering from a serious illness or surgery,
- Take blood pressure regulating medications or heart medications,
- Wear a pacemaker or other implanted electronic device.

■ **Choose the Right Load**

Avoid excessive demands

It is crucial to find the right amount of exercise stimulus for your body. So far, the lack of movement has led to your body being underchallenged. Too strong sudden physical demands, however, can overstrain the body. Both under- and overchallenge are harmful. As a rule of thumb, while exercising you should be able to talk to somebody on the side. If you want to determine the training intensity more precisely, you can refer to the pulse rate (heart rate, HR) as an easily measurable variable for the correct load.

■ How Do I Take My Pulse?

To do this, you need a watch with a second counter. You can feel your pulse on your wrist, carotid artery, or directly on your heart and count how many times your pulse beats in 10 s. Then take this number times 6. This gives you the number of beats per minute. It is easier and more reliable to measure your pulse using a heart rate monitor, which you can purchase at sporting goods stores or medical supply stores. To determine the correct training load, you need to know your maximum heart rate (MHR). To estimate your MHR, simply subtract your age in years from 220.

Maximum heart rate (MHR) = 220 minus age

Based on your maximum heart rate, you can use the percentages below to calculate your training heart rate for different training goals.

50–60% of MHR = training to stabilize health

Exercising at a heart rate of 50–60% of your MHR promotes health stabilization. This is light training (e.g. fast walking), but already provides health benefits.

60–70% of MHR = training to activate fat metabolism

When you increase your heart rate to 60–70% of your MHR, you are doing a workout to activate fat metabolism. This heart rate is good for fitness and promotes weight loss.

70–85% of the MHR = training to improve fitness

Training at 70–85% of your MHR is suitable for improving fitness. Here the training is already more strenuous, but it is worth it—provided you enjoy it.

More than 85% of the MHR = Anaerobic zone

Anaerobic training means that carbohydrates are metabolized for energy under oxygen-deficient conditions. This leads to over-acidification of the muscles (lactate formation) and can force you to stop exercising prematurely. Physical training at more than 85% of MHR is only **suitable** for competitive athletes, but **not** for the health athlete.

◘ Table 8.3 provides an overview of the aerobic heart rate target zones in heartbeats per minute, staggered by age (◘ Table 8.3).

■ Take Breaks, But Do It Right!

Especially at the beginning of your training, you will not be able to run or swim for 20 min at a time. If you just start running as a beginner, you will most likely have to stop after only a few minutes, exhausted. This will be frustrating for you and will not provide any health benefits. Instead, it is important to take enough short walking breaks in between to prevent overexertion. It is important to note that the break time should be about one-third shorter than the exertion time. This allows you to recover, but prevents you from returning to your pre-

■ Table 8.3 Training pulse rates for different age groups and training goals

Act	MHF (220 – Age)	Stable health 50–60% of MHR	Active fat metabolism 60–70% of MHR	Improved fitness 70–85% of MHR
25	195	97–117	117–136	136–165
30	190	95–114	114–133	133–161
35	185	92–11	111–129	129–157
40	180	90–108	108–126	126–153
45	175	87–105	105–122	122–148
50	170	85–102	102–119	119–144
55	165	82–99	99–115	115–140
60	160	80–96	96–112	112–136
65	155	77–93	93–108	108–131

8

exercise level. With these breaks you can last 20 min even as a beginner! In jogging, for example, this could look like this for a total 20 min:

Week 1:	Alternate 2 min running – 1 min walking break
Week 2:	Alternate 3 min walking – 1 min walking break
Week 3:	Alternate 4 min walking – 1 min walking break
etc.	

You will increasingly be able to run for more minutes and take fewer breaks.

■ **Increase the Duration First, then the Intensity!**
When you start an exercise activity, first work on increasing the duration so that you can sustain the activity for at least 20 min at moderate intensity. Only then gradually start to increase the intensity, for example, run or swim faster.

■ **Only Regular Exercise Keeps You fit!**
Remember, only regular physical activity brings long-lasting benefits. Irregular physical activity only brings a short-term improvement in physical and mental well-being. For sport to work, it should be done regularly, preferably 3 times a week and then preferably for 20 min or longer each time.

■ **Do Not Forget to Warm Up!**

Warming up before the actual sporting activity helps to make muscles and joints flexible and loose and prevents injuries. Overall, this prepares the transition from rest to exercise.

■ **Drink Plenty of Fluids!**

The sporting activity causes you to sweat. This causes your body to lose fluid. It is essential that you compensate for this fluid loss. So drink plenty after every sporting activity.

> **The Best News at the End**
> Very soon after you have started your endurance training, you will notice the first positive changes. Immediately after training you will feel invigorated, refreshed, or pleasantly relaxed. You will notice improvements in your fitness sooner than expected and feel more balanced and stronger overall. That is the good news: your body will immediately reward you for the exercise you give it!

For Acute Cases:
The 4-Step-Strategy

Contents

© Springer-Verlag GmbH Germany, part of Springer Nature 2022
G. Kaluza, *Calm and Confident Under Stress*, https://doi.org/10.1007/978-3-662-64440-9_9

9

Do you know this? You have experienced something nice in the evening, you have slept well and start the new day refreshed. You have pre-planned your day with sufficient time buffers and are confident that you will successfully master the challenges of the day. In short, your regenerative (enjoyment, sleep), instrumental (scheduling), and mental stress management (confidence) are working. And then, all of a sudden, you get stuck in a jam. That can take a while. Or your train is late, so you probably would not make it to your first appointment on time. Or the school calls while you are already having your first client meeting. Your son has injured himself and needs to be picked up. Or your boss tells you that you have to cover for a colleague who is sick on an important matter. You can forget your nice plan. Or you discover, while you are already on your way, that you have left the front door key stuck from the inside. Your daughter, who is coming home from school before you, will therefore not be able to get into the apartment. Or ... what comes to your mind?

These are some examples of acute stress situations. Situations that we can get into, that are unpredictable, that can never be completely avoided, no matter how well we have planned stress management in advance. Surely you know similar acute situations from your professional and private everyday life. These situations immediately activate the biological stress program: the heart pounds, we start to sweat, the stomach contracts, the muscles tense. Emotional arousal, fear, anger, perhaps rage rise. However, this physical and emotional activation is not really helpful in most cases. Fighting or fleeing are not realistic options. Instead, in such acute stressful situations, it is important not to be overwhelmed by the rising arousal, to maintain or regain control, and to keep a cool head in order to be able to recognize and take action options that may still exist. In this chapter, I will introduce you to a strategy that aims to do just that. It consists of four deliberate steps (◘ Fig. 9.1).

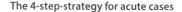

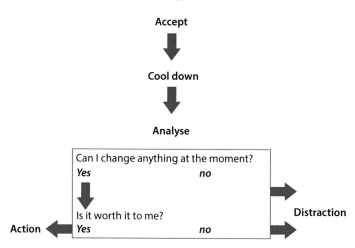

Fig. 9.1 The 4-step-strategy for acute cases

9.1 **Accept**

This is the first step of the strategy. Acceptance here means accepting the situation, the traffic jam, the train delay, the son's injury, the boss's additional order, the forgotten front door key, etc. as a fact that has occurred and cannot be changed. However, that does not mean helplessly surrendering to the situation. Acceptance is not the same as passively enduring or tolerating the situation (see ▶ Sect. 7.1). Rather, acceptance puts an end to the fruitless agonizing over what has happened, and it protects us from doing (or not doing) certain things out of acute agitation that would only make the situation worse than it already is. Acceptance helps us to focus our attention on the possibilities for action that may still exist, that we may still be able to take, not to undo the situation that has occurred, but to limit its consequences.

Acceptance requires a conscious decision. By consciously deciding in favour of acceptance and thus against struggling, we take a first decisive step out of the victim role and regain control over the situation.

9.2 Cooling Down

This second step of the strategy is aimed at getting a grip on excessive arousal in an acute stress situation, when one is "out of one's mind", wants to "go ballistic" or "no longer knows where front and back are". The point here is to collect oneself, to find one's own centre (again), to keep one's feet on the ground, and to keep a clear head. How can this succeed? Again, it is important to make a conscious decision for cooling down (and thus against getting caught up in the excitement). The cooling down itself can be achieved—depending on the situation—in very different ways. Sometimes just a few deep breaths are enough—perhaps at an open window. Others it helps to drink a glass of water or run cold water over your hands. Exercise can also help cool you down. Standing up, walking around the room a few steps while consciously putting your feet on the floor, even stretching vigorously or shaking yourself once can help "blow off steam". If you have trained a relaxation technique (▶ Chap. 8) well, you can now also use it in an acute stress situation and "shut yourself down" with it.

9.3 Analyse

If we succeed in finding an accepting attitude in an acute stress situation and in regulating the rising physical and emotional arousal, then we have already gained a lot. Outwardly, nothing has changed in the situation, but we have changed. By consciously and decisively accepting and cooling down, we have taken the reins back into our own hands. In the next, the third step of the strategy, it is then a matter of taking a short moment to come to a conscious and quick assessment of our own options for action. We do this by asking ourselves, "Is there anything I can do right now?" When we recognize our own options for action, we assess them in terms of effort and benefit: "Is it worth it to me?" This second assessment is necessary to counter the danger of rash or overly elaborate actions ("making too much fuss"). You do not have to take every identified course of action right away. Instead of lapsing into blind actionism, it is sometimes wiser to wait and see, to let things rest or come to you.

9.4 Action or Distraction

The result of the brief analysis in the previous step then leads either to taking specific action to influence the current situation or its consequences ("action"), or to doing something to distance oneself from the current situation and take care of one's own well-being ("distraction"). Either you take care of the situation, or you take care of yourself. Which possibilities of distraction or which possibilities of action there are in each case, depends course to a large extent on the concrete situation. Distraction can be, for example, through music, through reading, through pleasant thoughts, through watching other people, and so on. Direct actions can be, for example, drawing boundaries and saying "no", delegating tasks or seeking support, rearranging appointments, or rescheduling tasks at short notice.

These are the 4 steps of the acute case strategy. If you would like to use this strategy in your everyday life, then memorize its four steps very well and play through the strategy several times in your mind using past and possible future acute stress situations (▶ Box 9.1). The four steps should become second nature to you so that you can actually call them up in an acute situation.

> **Box 9.1: Exercise: Trying Out the 4-Step-Strategy Mentally**
> Recall as accurately as possible an acute stressful situation that you have recently encountered. Put yourself back into the situation and recall your physical, emotional, and mental stress reactions at the time. And then imagine yourself using the 4-step-strategy in that situation. Go through this strategy in your mind—step by step. At each step, be very clear about what you are specifically doing or thinking in order to implement each step, and feel how this affects your physical and emotional arousal. Repeat this mental play through of the 4-step-strategy several times in order to memorize the 4 steps as deeply as possible.

Finding Your Own Way

Contents

© Springer-Verlag GmbH Germany, part of Springer Nature 2022
G. Kaluza, *Calm and Confident Under Stress*, https://doi.org/10.1007/978-3-662-64440-9_10

10.1   The 3 × 4 of Stress Competence

In the previous chapters of this book, you learned about the three pillars of personal stress competence. For each of these three areas of competence, I have presented you with four basic stress management strategies. In the following checklist, you will find a concise summary of these 3 × 4 strategies for stress management (◻ Fig. 10.1). Please use the list to check in which areas your competences are already well developed today and with regard to which areas you would like to develop further in the future.

10

Checklist: The 3 x 4 of stress competence				

In this checklist you will find a brief summary of essential strategies for personal stress management. Please use the list to check in which areas your competences are already well developed today and in which areas you would like to develop further in the future.

I would like to change something in this area...

These statements apply to me...
5 = completely, 4 = mostly, 3 = partly, partly, 2 = hardly, 1 = not at all
Please enter the appropriate number!

			Yes	No	?
1. Instrumental stress competence					
1.1 I keep myself professionally up to date. I regularly take part in further training. I like to learn from others and see myself as a "learner".					
1.2 I maintain my social network. I receive sufficient support from others. I have at least one trusted person with whom I can let myself go.					
1.3 I respect my boundaries. I represent my interests to others. If necessary, I say "no", delegate tasks or ask others for support.					
1.4 I have a positive vision for the future and clear goals. I set priorities. I plan my time accordingly and pay attention to my personal performance curve.					
Total Domain 1					
2. Mental stress competence					
2.1 For me, demands and difficulties are part of life. I face them with an accepting attitude.					
2.2 I see demands or difficulties as a positive challenge. I assess them realistically and maintain an inner distance.					

◻ **Fig. 10.1** The 3 × 4 of stress competence

I would like to change something in this area...

These statements apply to me...
5 = completely, 4 = mostly, 3 = partly, partly, 2 = hardly, 1 = not at all
Please enter the appropriate number!

		Yes	No	?
2.3 I have a strong confidence in my own competences. I am aware of my strengths and I am confident that I can cope with new challenges and difficulties.				
2.4 I am aware of my personal stress amplifiers. I work specifically on my personal development. I defuse my personal stress amplifiers by actively trying out new behaviour, e.g. allowing mistakes, relinquishing control or asking for help.				
Total Area 2				
3. Regenerative stress competence				
3.1 I provide regular breaks. I organise my holidays according to my recreational needs. I have a deep and restful sleep.				
3.2 In my free time, I actively provide a counterbalance to my work. I do activities that are fun for me and I enjoy pleasant things.				
3.3 I have mastered a relaxation method that enables me to relax physically and switch off mentally.				
3.4 I exercise regularly and make sure I get plenty of exercise in my daily life.				
Total Domain 3				

❓ Evaluation questions:
  ▬ Which pillars of stress competence are strong, which are less strong?
  ▬ In which areas would I like to develop my stress competence in the future?
  ▬ What next steps will I take to expand my stress competence?

◘ Fig. 10.1 (continued)

10.2 A Word in Conclusion

» Even the longest journey begins with the first lifting of the foot. (Lao Tzu, legendary Chinese philosopher, 6th century B.C.)

Dear Reader,

Attitudes and behaviours that have often grown over many years and shape the way we deal with stress today do not change overnight, certainly not by themselves. The will to work on yourself, time, and patience are necessary investments in your personal process towards a healthier way of dealing with the stressors of everyday life.

Please heed the following advice:

— Do not take on too much at once. Set yourself manageable realistic goals and plan individual concrete steps.

— Always visualize your advantages that you want to achieve and will achieve. This will help you overcome obstacles that arise.

— Realize that setbacks can occur in any attempt to change behaviour. Setbacks are normal. Do not be discouraged and be patient with yourself.

— Together it is often easier. Courses on stress management are offered by health insurance companies, adult education centres, and other adult education institutions. There you will find competent support and the backing of a group of like-minded people.

— I wish you much success on your personal path to more serenity, well-being, and health.

Sincerely
Your
Gert Kaluza

Supplementary Information

© Springer-Verlag GmbH Germany, part of Springer Nature 2022

G. Kaluza, *Calm and Confident Under Stress*, https://doi.org/10.1007/978-3-662-64440-9

Literature

Allmer H (1996) Erholung und Gesundheit. Grundlagen, Ergebnisse und Maßnahmen. Hogrefe, Göttingen

Antonovsky A (1988) Unraveling the mystery of health. How people manage stress and stay well. Jossey-Bass, San Francisco

Bandura A (1977) Self-efficacy: toward a unifying theory of behavioral change. Psychol Rev 84:191–215

Bauer J (2005) Das Gedächtnis des Körpers. Wie Beziehungen und Lebensstile unsere Gene steuern. 3. Aufl. Piper, München

Benkert O (2005) Stressdepression. Die neue Volkskrankheit und was man dagegen tun kann. Beck, München

Bernstein DA, Borkovec TD (1990) Entspannungstraining. Handbuch der progressiven Muskelentspannung. Pfeiffer, München

Bouchard C, Shepard RJ, Stephens T, Sutton JR, McPherson BD (1991) Exercise, fitness and health—a consensus of current knowledge. Human Kinetics Books, Champaign/Ill

Brechtel C (1994) Muskuläres Tiefentraining—neue Wege zur Entspannung. psychotop, Durbach

Burisch M (1994) Das Burnout-Syndrom. 2. Aufl. Springer, Heidelberg

Buske-Kirschbaum A, Kirschbaum C, Hellhammer D (1990) Psychoneuroimmunologie. In: Schwarzer R (Hrsg) Gesundheitspsychologie. Ein Lehrbuch. Hogrefe, Göttingen, S 35–44

Cannon WB (1929) Bodily changes in pain, hunger, fear and rage. Appleton, New York

Covey SR, Merill AR, Merrill RR (1997) Der Weg zum Wesentlichen. Zeitmanagement der vierten Generation. Campus, Frankfurt am Main

Eberspächer H (1998) Ressource Ich. Der ökonomische Umgang mit Streß. Hanser, München

Frankl VE (1981) Die Sinnfrage in der Psychotherapie. Piper, München

Frankl VE (1994) Logotherapie und Existenzanalyse. Texte aus sechs Jahrzehnten. Quintessenz, München

Fuchs E, Flügge G (2001) Psychosoziale Belastung hinterlässt Spuren im Gehirn. Z Med Psychol 10:99–105

Hamm A (1993) Progressive Muskelentspannung. In: Vaitl D, Petermann F (Hrsg) Handbuch der Entspannungsverfahren. Band 1: Grundlagen und Methoden. Psychologie Verlags Union, Weinheim, S 245–264

Hoffmann F (2005) "Gönne Dich Dir selbst"—Monastische Burnout-Prophylaxe. Deutsches Pfarrerblatt 8:35

Holmes TH, Rahe RH (1967) The Social Readjustment Rating Scale. J Psychosom Res 11:213–218

Hüther G (1997) Biologie der Angst. Wie aus Stress Gefühle werden. Vandenhoeck & Ruprecht, Göttingen

Jacobson E (1993) Entspannung als Therapie. Progressive Relaxation in Theorie und Praxis. Pfeiffer, München

Jansen R (2000) Arbeitsbelastungen und Arbeitsbedingungen. In: Badura B, Litsch M, Vetter C (Hrsg) Fehlzeiten-Report 1999. Psychische Belastung am Arbeitsplatz. Springer, Berlin, Heidelberg, S 5–30

Kaluza G (1996) Belastungsbewältigung und Gesundheit—Theoretische Perspektiven und empirische Befunde. Z Med Psychol 5:147–155

Kaluza G (1999) Optimismus und Gesundheit: Gibt es eine salutogene Konstruktion subjektiver Realität? Psychomed 11:51–57

Kaluza G (2004) Stressbewältigung. Trainingsmanual zur psychologischen Gesundheitsförderung. Springer, Heidelberg

Kaluza G, Vögele C (1999) Stress und Stressbewältigung. In: Flor H, Birbaumer N, Hahlweg K (Hrsg) Enzyklopädie der Psychologie, Themenbereich D Praxisgebiete, Serie II Klinische Psychologie, Band 3 Grundlagen der Verhaltensmedizin. Hogrefe, Göttingen, S 331–388

Kaluza G, Basler HD, Simon G, Schmidt-Trucksäß A, Büchler G (1998) Wohlbefinden und kardiovaskuläre Fitness bei Teilnehmern eines laktatgesteuerten Ausdauertrainings. Zeitschrift für Gesundheitspsychologie 6:33–36

Kaluza G, Keller S, Basler HD (2001) Beanspruchungsregulation durch Sport?—Zusammenhänge zwischen wahrgenommener Arbeitsbelastung, sportlicher Aktivität und psychophysischem Wohlbefinden. Zeitschrift für Gesundheitspsychologie 9:26–31

Karasek RA, Theorell T (1990) Healthy work: stress, productivity and the restruction of working life. Basic Books, New York

Karasek RA, Bauer D, Marxer A, Theorell T (1981) Job decision latitude, job demands and cardiovascular disease: a prospective study of Swedish men. Am J Public Health 71:694–705

Kirschbaum C, Hellhammer D (1999) Hypothalamus-Hypophysen-Nebennierenrindenachse. In: Birbaumer N, Frey D, Kuhl J, Prinz W, Weinert FE (Hrsg) Enzyklopädie der Psychologie: Themenbereich C Theorie und Forschung, Serie I Biologische Psychologie, Band 3 Psychoendokrinologie und Psychoimmunologie. Hogrefe, Göttingen, S 79–140

Koppenhöfer E (2004) Kleine Schule des Genießens. Pabst, Lengerich

Lazarus RS (1966) Psychological stress and the coping process. McGraw-Hill, New York

Lazarus RS, Launier R, (1981) Streßbezogene Transaktionen zwischen Person und Umwelt. In: Nitsch JR (Hrsg) Stress. Theorien, Untersuchungen, Maßnahmen. Huber, Bern, S 213–259

Ledoux JE (1999) Das Gedächtnis für Angst. Spektrum der Wissenschaft Dossier 3:16–23

Linehan M (1996) Trainingsmanual zur Dialektisch-Behavioralen Therapie der Borderline-Persönlichkeitsstörung. Cip-Medien, München

Lohmann-Haislah A (2012) Stressreport Deutschland 2012. Psychische Anforderungen, Ressourcen und Befinden. Bundesanstalt für Arbeitsschutz und Arbeitsmedizin, Dortmund

Lutz R (1993) Genußtraining. In: Linden M, Hautzinger M (Hrsg) Verhaltenstherapie. Techniken und Einzelverfahren. Springer, Berlin, S 155–159

Maslach C, Leiter MP (2001) Die Wahrheit über Burnout—Stress am Arbeitsplatz und was Sie dagegen tun können. Springer, Wien, New York

Matyssek, AK (2007) Führungsfaktor Gesundheit. So bleiben Führungskräfte und Mitarbeiter gesund. Gabal, Offenbach

Mentzel G (1979) Über die Arbeitssucht. Z Psychosom Med Psychoanal 25:115–127

Menz W, Dunkel W, Kratzer N (2011) Leistung und Leiden. Neue Steuerungsformen von Leistung und ihre Belastungswirkungen. In: Kratzer N, Dunkel W, Becker K, Hinrichs S (Hrsg) Arbeit und Gesundheit im Konflikt—Analysen und Ansätze für ein partizipatives Gesundheitsmanagement. edition sigma, Berlin, S 143–198

Nemeroff C (1999) Neurobiologie der Angst. Spektrum der Wisssenschaft Dossier 3:24–31

O'Leary A (1984) Self-efficacy and health. Behav Res Ther 23:437–451

Poppelreuter S (1997) Arbeitssucht. Psychologie Verlags Union, Weinheim

Röhrle B (1994) Soziale Netzwerke und soziale Unterstützung. Psychologie Verlags Union, Weinheim

Rudow B (2004) Das gesunde Unternehmen. Oldenbourg, München

Rugulies R, Siegrist J (2002) Soziologische Aspekte der Entstehung und des Verlaufes der chronischen Herzkrankheit. Soziale Ungleichverteilung der Erkrankung und chronische Distress-Erfahrungen im Erwerbsleben. VAS, Frankfurt am Main

Sapolsky RM (1996) Why stress is bad for your brain. Science 273:749–750

Schedlowski M (1994) Stress, Hormone und zelluläre Immunfunktionen. Spektrum Akademischer Verlag, Heidelberg

Schlicht W (1993) Psychische Gesundheit durch Sport? Realität oder Wunsch: Eine Meta-Analyse. Zeitschrift für Gesundheitspsychologie 1:65–81

Schmid W (1998) Philosophie der Lebenskunst. Suhrkamp, Heidelberg

Schultz JH (1979) Das autogene Training. Konzentrative Selbstentspannung. Thieme, Stuttgart

Schulz von Thun F (1989) Miteinander reden 2.Stile, Werte und Persönlichkeitsentwicklung. Rowohlt, Reinbek

Schwarzer R (1993) Defensiver und funktionaler Optimismus als Bedingungen für Gesundheitsverhalten. Zeitschrift für Gesundheitspsychologie 1:7–31

Schwarzer R, Leppin A (1989) Sozialer Rückhalt und Gesundheit. Eine Meta-Analyse. Hogrefe, Göttingen

Seiwert LJ (2001) Wenn Du es eilig hast, gehe langsam. Das neue Zeitmanagement in einer beschleunigten Welt. Sieben Schritte zur Zeitsouveränität und Effektivität. Campus, Frankfurt am Main

Seligman M (1979) Erlernte Hilflosigkeit. Urban & Schwarzenberg, München

Selye H (1936) A syndrome produced by diverse nocious agents. Nature 138:32

Selye H (1981) Geschichte und Grundzüge des Stresskonzeptes. In: Nitsch JR (Hrsg) Stress. Theorien, Untersuchungen, Maßnahmen. Huber, Bern, S 163–187

Siegrist J (1996) Soziale Krisen und Gesundheit. Hogrefe, Göttingen

Siegrist J, Dragano N (2008) Psychosoziale Belastungen und Erkrankungsrisiken im Erwerbsleben. Befunde aus internationalen Studien zum Anforderungs-Kontroll-Modell und zum Modell beruflicher Gratifikationskrisen. Bundesgesundheitsblatt 51:S 305–312

Theorell T, Harms Ringdahl K, Ahlberg Hutten G, Westin B (1991) Psychosocial job factors and symptoms from the locomotor system—a multicausal analysis. Scand J Rehabil Med 23:165–173

Uvnäs-Moberg K, Petersson M (2005) Oxytocin, ein Vermittler von Antistress, Wohlbefinden, sozialer Interaktion, Wachstum und Heilung. Z Psychosom Med Psychother 51:57–80

Vahtera J et al (2004) Organisational downsizing, sickness absence, and mortality: 10-town prospective cohort study. Br Med J 328:555–560

Watzlawick P (1988) Anleitung zum Unglücklichsein. Piper, München

Zulley J, Knab B (2002) Die kleine Schlafschule. Herder, Freiburg

Index

Printed in the United States
by Baker & Taylor Publisher Services